PRINCIPLES OF
EXPERIMENTAL
PSYCHOLOGY

Founded by C. K. Ogden

The International Library of Psychology

INDIVIDUAL DIFFERENCES
In 21 Volumes

PRINCIPLES OF EXPERIMENTAL PSYCHOLOGY

HENRI PIÉRON

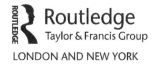

Routledge
Taylor & Francis Group

LONDON AND NEW YORK

First published in 1929 by
Kegan Paul, Trench, Trubner & Co., Ltd.
2 Park Square, Milton Park, Abingdon, Oxfordshire OX14 4RN
711 Third Avenue, New York, NY 10017

First issued in paperback 2014

Routledge is an imprint of the Taylor and Francis Group, an informa business

© 1929 Henri Piéron, Translated by J B Miner

All rights reserved. No part of this book may be reprinted or reproduced
or utilized in any form or by any electronic, mechanical, or other means,
now known or hereafter invented, including photocopying
and recording, or in any information storage or retrieval system, without
permission in writing from the publishers.

The publishers have made every effort to contact authors/copyright holders
of the works reprinted in the *International Library of Psychology*.
This has not been possible in every case, however, and we would
welcome correspondence from those individuals/companies
we have been unable to trace.

These reprints are taken from original copies of each book. In many cases
the condition of these originals is not perfect. The publisher has gone to
great lengths to ensure the quality of these reprints, but wishes to point
out that certain characteristics of the original copies will, of necessity, be
apparent in reprints thereof.

British Library Cataloguing in Publication Data
A CIP catalogue record for this book
is available from the British Library

Principles of Experimental Psychology
ISBN 978-0415-21066-9
Individual Differences: 21 Volumes
ISBN 0415-21130-1
The International Library of Psychology: 204 Volumes
ISBN 0415-19132-7

ISBN 13: 978-1-138-88254-6 (pbk)
ISBN 13: 978-0-415-21066-9 (hbk)

CONTENTS

CONTENTS

PART FOUR

PART FIVE

PART SIX

PREFACE

ACCORDING to academic tradition this volume would be a section of philosophy, but it is really concerned with a branch of biology. It sets forth the principles generally stated in connection with the scientific study of the mental functions of living beings, having more especially to do with normal civilized man, who interests us in practical life.

Instead of a simple arrangement of facts, laws and measurements, the reader will find a general exposition of mental functioning such as may be disentangled from the results hitherto obtained, with an appeal to examples of definite accomplishment. This provisional synthesis will undoubtedly appear very unlike the familiar descriptions set forth by classical psychology, from which it is difficult to free one's self in spite of their artificial character.

In order to retrace the work of a science in a few pages, it has been necessary to dispense with the encumbering apparatus of citations and references. Only exceptionally will a name be cited in connection with a fact or a discovery. Otherwise it would have been necessary to load the text with too great a number of authors. Behind a phrase, a line, or a note, have very often been concealed much splendid work, discussion and computation, of which only the summarized result appears.

In order not to make the bibliographical index a volume in itself, it has been necessary to limit it to a few general works. To choose a few among the works bearing upon particular problems would have been too arbitrary and unjust. Facts necessarily take on an independent life very quickly, so that the names of those who have discovered them are forgotten. If one tried to-day, in a chapter of physics, to attribute the accepted principles to their true authors, it would be possible to do so for only a few discoveries of the first rank and a few important laws.

Finally, the brief historical suggestions of the Introduction stop at the time when the scientific movement in psychology had become general, thanks to the convergent efforts of numerous scientists of all countries. For the most part these are still living. Among those in France we must at least cite Alfred Binet, Georges Dumas, Pierre Janet, and Edouard Toulouse for the importance and the fruitfulness of their work.

H. Piéron.

PRINCIPLES OF EXPERIMENTAL PSYCHOLOGY

INTRODUCTION

A. Historical.

SCIENCE and philosophy have been for a long time confounded. What characterizes science is the appeal to verification, the subordination of theories to facts, in short, the experimental attitude ; while philosophy is satisfied with internal logical coherence and limits itself progressively to problems which cannot be submitted to experimental control.

The Greeks, who were the first seekers after knowledge, commenced by ignoring this distinction between the empirical and the logical, and by considering all problems in the same way. Sometimes they gave the logical method first place, sometimes the empirical. After Plato, who took refuge in a world of ideas, came Aristotle, who opened people's eyes to the world of nature. In his effort towards universal science—still, of course, thoroughly penetrated with metaphysics—he viewed psycho-physiology as standing at the side of physiology and physics. Moreover, he collected numerous facts which were later taken over by scientific psychology. Not till we come to Descartes do we find scientific observations concerning mental functions, although they are expressed in a language filled with conceptions which to-day raise a smile. They must be considered, however, in relation to the time when they were written.

Then, with the development of an empirical philosophy, the experimental method was accepted as valuable for psychology as well as for all other branches of knowledge. This philosophy was represented by Hobbes, Locke, Hume, Reid, Hamilton and J. S. Mill. But only in establishing the laws of the association of ideas did psychology disengage itself from philosophy. For Kant, who gave science its place in the system of knowledge, there was no scientific psychology possible. The positivism of Auguste Comte left the phenomena of consciousness outside the important branches of knowledge, the social being superimposed directly upon the biological.

Modern philosophy has continued to discuss the methodological problem of psychology, asking to what extent the phenomenon of consciousness is accessible to the experimental method. Its object is to understand the nature of the agreement between the series of subjective events, which one knows by introspection, and the objective events, which are the same for one's self as for others, and are known through the organs of sense. Postponing for a time the definite solution of this problem, it is content to affirm a " psycho-physical parallelism."

During these discussions of its legitimacy and methods, however, the science of psychology was establishing itself, and had for a long time been developing in a manner entirely independent of philosophical speculation.

It might be thought that psychology would at first develop as a science among physicians and then among naturalists. But in reality medicine has been impregnated with *a priori* concepts, from which it has had difficulty in freeing itself even in our time. It has been more philosophical and speculative than scientific and empirical. The naturalistic theorists, while giving an important place to facts, were also preoccupied above all in constructing explanations which in general elude verification and remain, for the most part, purely philosophical (Lamarck, Darwin, Spencer).

Experimental psychology in reality was born from physics. It was among research men, accustomed to the requirements of scientific method, that experimentation has been extended from external phenomena to the mental processes implied by the knowledge of these phenomena. The extension was often unperceived from the fact that the physicists for a long time believed that they were studying physical processes when making their investigations on the psycho-physiological phenomena which these processes, then badly understood, aroused. Sound was studied before the vibratory phenomena which arouse it. Light is still sometimes confounded with the particular radiations which are able to give birth to it. In studying the phenomena of light and sound the physicists were very naturally led to study hearing and vision.

Joseph Sauveur, of La Flèche (1663–1716), himself almost completely deaf, demonstrated, on individuals endowed with a good musical ear, the existence of difference tones when the frequency of beats became sufficiently great, and established the possibility of a dissociation of overtones in audition, showing that there was not a fusion in the auditory apparatus of simultaneous sounds of different pitch. This differs from the fusion that occurs in the visual apparatus.

Philip de la Hire, of Paris (1640–1718) drew attention to the phenomena of after-images with their characteristic succession of colours, influenced by the backgrounds on which the images are projected.

In 1765, Chevalier d'Arcy measured the persistence of certain luminous impressions, fixing thirteen or fifteen-hundredths of a second as that for the image of heated carbon. The adaptation to darkness, with the correlative increase in the sensibility to light, was studied by W. Herschell (1730–1822), the astronomer of Hanover. He likewise noted, what had already been noticed by one of the Cassini, that in a feeble light it is not the centre of the retina which has the greatest sensitivity, but a peripheral region. The observation of the feeble satellites of Saturn requires a fixation of the eye at a certain distance from the position of the satellites.

The Italian physicist Venturi measured the normal visual field. Ptolemy, following Heliodorus of Larissa, had described it as a right-angled cone, in connection with his penetrating study of the exploratory function of the eye in the construction of visual images.

The first psychological law, the empirical law named after Weber, for which the metaphysics of Fechner won so much fame, the fundamental law of psycho-physics, is due to a French physicist, Bouguer (1698–1758). It is found set forth in the *Traité d'Optique sur la Gradation de la Lumière*. In order to be perceived, a variation of light must be a constant proportion (a sixty-fourth) of the original light. Another French physicist, Masson (1806–1860), confirmed the work of Bouguer in 1845, and expressed it by saying, "The sensibility of the eye is independent of the intensity of the light."

The astronomers, on their side, classified the stars according to their luminosity in steps which were judged equally distant. They established the fact that the series of stellar magnitudes corresponded to variations of luminosity in a sensibly constant proportion, in accordance with the law of Bouguer-Masson. W. Herschell found that the fourth magnitude corresponded in actual brightness to about a sixteenth of that of the first magnitude, the sixth to a value of very nearly a sixty-fourth. The rate of the progression is, moreover, exact, and measured by $1/2 \cdot 5$.[1] (The sixth magnitude corresponds to a brightness a hundred times less than the first.)

In the course of the more systematic researches of the German physiologist Weber (1851), the fundamental law of psycho-physics was formulated as a first approximation, of course.[2]

The relations of the steps of tonal sensation to the frequencies of vibration of the sound waves was the object of the researches of Euler (1739), then of Herbart (1807),

---

[1] The exponents of Steinheil (1837), of Stumpfer, of Johnson, of Pogson (1856), are : 2·702, 2·519, 2·158, 2·400.

[2] It is curious that the formula adopted by Fechner was at first proposed in the much more complex domain of morals. Bernoulli (1738) and later Laplace (1749–1827), in the *Traité analytique des Probabilités*, in the course of mathematical considerations, suggested that this relation was found between moral fortune (happiness) and physical fortune (riches), according to which happiness increased as the logarithm of riches.

and Drobisch (1846). Délezenne (1827), the physicist of Lille, showed by the sonometer that the finest differential sensibility for pitch corresponded very nearly to a half or a quarter of a musical " comma."

The systematization of research on vision and audition was due to the genius of Helmholtz (1821–1894), who was at the same time a physiologist and a physicist. This constituted, under the form of the psycho-physiology of the senses, the first branch of experimental psychology.

It is particularly to the astronomers that the credit is due for the foundation of what is sometimes called " psycho-chronometry."

As early as 1795 the astronomer at Greenwich, Maskelyne, observed the mistakes of individuals in the notation of the simultaneity between the apparent position of a star with reference to the thread of the telescope and a beat of a pendulum. In 1820 Bessel systematically studied this " personal equation," considering the difficulties in appreciating the simultaneity between heterogeneous impressions. When, in order to avoid these difficulties, the apparent passage of the star behind the thread was registered by a graphic reaction, new errors appeared, due to the retardation, after the sensory stimulus, of the movement called forth. The study of " reaction times," so named by Exner (1879), was thus introduced.[1]

In the medical observation of diseases of the brain, too, the objective spirit and the experimental tendency soon made progress; but pathological psychology constitutes a sufficiently developed branch of scientific psychology to allow it its own autonomy without annexing it to experimental psychology proper.

We will only note, on the borderline of the pathological and the normal, the researches bearing on the mental effects of certain toxins, in particular the analysis of the

---

[1] In the numerical notations, which the astronomers who gave the signals would also make, called " decimal equations," it was curious that different individuals had preferences for certain numbers which brought about systematic errors of notation.

exhilarating effect of nitrous oxide, or "laughing gas," by Humphry Davy as early as 1799.

Finally physiology, when it became an independent science, turned its attention to the sense organs and the functions of the nervous system. It was thus led in the nineteenth century, to the study of the mental processes by the method of objective experiment. The physiologist Weber (1795–1878) began, especially in the perception of weights, the quantitative researches on the sensitivity to differences which were to give birth to the psycho-physical theory of Fechner (1860).

It is to the psycho-physics of Fechner (1801–1887), who was a physician in Leipzig, where he was a student of Weber, before he taught physics, that we trace the first manifestation of scientific autonomy given by experimental psychology.

But, in seeking to establish numerical relations between physical phenomena and the processes of consciousness, Fechner was still involved in the field of metaphysics.

Psychological experimentation proceeds much more truly from Helmholtz. After some medical and biological studies, his thesis being on the ganglia of invertebrates, Helmholtz accepted an independent chair of physiology in Heidelberg, the first in Germany. Having begun the study of the sensory processes of hearing and of vision, he gave himself up entirely to researches in psycho-physiology and physics, and soon passed to the chair of physics at Berlin (1871). But Helmholtz differed from Fechner by always remaining in the field of experimental science.

It is to a student of Helmholtz, Wundt (1832–1920), that we must properly ascribe the establishment of experimental psychology as a fully independent discipline. After his study of medicine and physics, Wundt continued at first the study of the psycho-physiology of the senses, while teaching physiology. In 1862 he published some contributions to the theory of sensory perception. He was not slow, however, to turn towards philosophy, as Fechner had also done. Appointed professor of philosophy at Leipzig (1875), he organized immediately a laboratory for psychological research, which was not recognized by the university until 1886. He gathered many students there, and directed the carrying out of numerous works published in the *Philosophische Studien*. This was founded in 1883 with the double tendency of philosophical speculation and the experimental spirit. The psychology of Wundt, set forth in his *Grundzüge der physiologischen Psychologie* (first edition, 1875 ; sixth edition, 1915), resulted in a compromise between the two tendencies. The other students of Helmholtz, like Exner (1846–1926), the physiologist of Vienna, and Hering (1834–1918), remained with advantage in the purely scientific field, but did not exert as much influence as Wundt.

From all sides the movement towards psychological research was planned and pursued by the effort sometimes of philosophers, sometimes of physiologists. Laboratories were created, periodicals founded, and results accumulated. While the legitimacy of the new science did not cease to be discussed for half a century, it little by little became a considerable edifice.

In 1879 G. Müller founded at Goettingen a laboratory of psycho-physics. Martius installed a laboratory of psychology at Bonn in 1888. The *Zeitschrift für Psychologie* began to be published by Ebbinghaus and Koenig in 1890.

In France the positive movement in psychology dates from the publication of *l'Intelligence* by Taine (1870), who derived his chief material from pathological sources. It was at Salpêtrière that the experimental spirit, still under the influence of pathology, developed through the initiative of Charcot (1825–1893). Binet, Pierre Janet, and Féré were his pupils. The philosopher Ribot (1839–1916) understood and set forth with admirable clarity the new position of psychology. In 1876 he founded the *Revue Philosophique*, which became the organ of the young school. The main features of the scientific movement in England (1870) and in Germany (1879) were made known, and Ribot began a series of remarkable

studies, the inspiration of which was still mainly pathological. The physiologist, Charles Richet, devoting
himself also to the scientific investigation of mental
processes, published among his first works, *Recherches
expérimentales et cliniques sur la sensibilité* (1877).[1] In
1887 he published a *Psychologie générale*, in which he
showed himself to be above all a philosopher, but disclosed very strongly his desire to apply the experimental
method especially to the most mysterious phenomena of
telepathy, somnambulism, etc.

Again it was a physiologist, Beaunis (1830–1925), who,
in connection with researches on hypnotism, pursued
psycho-physiological studies which were truly experimental; for example, those on the conditions of cerebral
activity. Giving up his chair at Nancy, he came to Paris
in 1889 to direct the first French laboratory,[2] while at the
Collège de France the chair of experimental psychology
was founded for Ribot in 1888 on the initiative of
Renan.

L'Année Psychologique was founded by Beaunis and
Binet, with the collaboration of Ribot, in 1893.

In Italy the anthropologist Sergi published, as early as
1873, the *Principles of Physiological Psychology*, and, in
December, 1889, he effected the organization of a laboratory at the University of Rome. In 1883 the psychiatrist
at Turin, Buccola, set forth in an excellent work, the
laws of time in the phenomena of thought. The psychia-

---

[1] In the introduction to this work, Richet declared : " Psychology
tends every day to become a more and more exact science. One can
foresee the time when it will be one of the most interesting branches of
physiology. . . ." He also proclaimed in it the necessity of a " rigorously experimental " method (p. 8).

[2] This was the laboratory of physiological psychology of the Sorbonne,
attached to the Section of Natural Sciences of the École pratique des
Hautes Études. It was soon after directed by Alfred Binet (1857–1911)
with Courtier and Philippe as regular collaborators and Victor Henri
as voluntary collaborator. Pierre Janet secured from Charcot the
foundation of a laboratory of psychology at Salpêtrière. In 1901 Ed.
Toulouse had attached to the École des Hautes Études a laboratory of
experimental psychology situated at the Asylum of Villejuif, with
Vaschide and Piéron as collaborators ; while, at the Asylum Sainte-
Anne the laboratory of psychology was connected with the chair of
mental diseases and had Georges Dumas for its chief.

trist Tamburini (1848–1919) undertook research and created a psychological laboratory at the asylum of Reggio Emilia in 1896.

In England the private and entirely independent initiative of Galton (1822-1892) organized experimental psychology in the applied field as a branch of anthropometry. Meanwhile the new psychology was taught by Ward (1843–1925) at Cambridge University, from 1882 onwards.

In the United States, Ladd (1842–1920) published his *Elements of Physiological Psychology* as early as 1887, the date of the founding of the *American Journal of Psychology* by Stanley Hall, a pupil of Wundt, who started the first American laboratory at Baltimore in 1885 at Johns Hopkins University. In 1888, Cattell, at the University of Pennsylvania in Philadelphia, occupied the first chair of experimental psychology. In 1890 William James (1840–1910) published his *Principles of Psychology*, which had considerable influence. The *Psychological Review* was established in 1893.

Everywhere, in the last quarter of the nineteenth century the new psychology was organized and developed.[1] By the beginning of the twentieth century, the period of organization was ended. In addition to speculative research, we find, in the line of investigation developed by Galton, some psychometric work intended for practical use.

B. *Purpose and Methods.*

To define the aim and the method of a science is the province not of science, but of philosophy. One might well abstain from treating this epistemological question.

[1] It may be further noted that, in Switzerland, Th. Flournoy (1854–1910), a student of Wundt, secured in 1891 at the University of Geneva the establishment of a laboratory and of a chair of experimental psychology, attached to the Faculty of Science and actually occupied by Ed. Claparède. In Denmark, Alfred Lehmann, former student of Wundt, founded a laboratory at Copenhagen and became professor in 1910. There might also be cited Tokarsky in Russia, the physicist Plateau in Belgium, etc.

General philosophy, in so far as it still occupies itself with psychology, faces this problem, the solution of which evidently is not affected by the facts or the laws discovered by experimental research. However, as the separation between philosophy and psychology has not been effected without allowing some connections to persist, one is warranted in not allowing psychologists to speak of their work without first justifying the right of their science to its existence, which one would nevertheless not contest as a fact. When we find the first theorists in experimental psychology, like Wundt or Ribot, striving to demonstrate the specific character of their science as the science of the phenomena of consciousness, at least of a "double-faced" phenomenon,[1] one understands how the question came to arise. The other natural sciences applied themselves to objective phenomena. Here was a science which pretended and affirmed that it set forth the laws of phenomena which were properly speaking subjective. For this reason Auguste Comte contested its right. But there was here, in reality, a gigantic illusion.

Let us consider this a little more closely. I look at a source of light provided from a monochromatic screen which permits a group of radiations of about 550 millimicrons to pass; I have a certain conscious impression, and I say to my neighbour, who is able to make note of it, that I have perceived "green"; I take note myself of

[1] Ribot, in his *English Psychology*, set forth his intention to show that psychology constituted an independent science, a natural science and not a purely descriptive natural history. He affirmed that "what is important is quantitative determination," and that "purely experimental psychology" would have for its object only "phenomena, their laws, and their immediate causes." But what phenomena? he inquired. In the *German Psychology of To-day*, he said that it had to do with the "nervous phenomena accompanying consciousness," concerning which psychology "found in man the type most easy to know, but which it should follow in all the animal series." He suggested that, "The nervous process as having a single face is for the physiologist, the nervous process as having a double face for the psychologist." Making his thought more precise, Ribot came still nearer to the position of Wundt, when he declared a little later, that between the science of the phenomena of consciousness and physiology there was the same relation as between the latter and the physico-chemical sciences.

this fact for future reference. My neighbour looks in his turn and declares that he also perceives green. I make a note of it. Then I utilize other screens under different conditions and I continue to note the conditions under which my neighbour and myself perceive green.

I thus study the sensation of green, which is for myself, I know by intimate experience, a conscious sensation. By analogy I admit that it is the same for my neighbour. But I have no means of knowing it, nor, in particular, of knowing whether his conscious impression is identical with mine. All I know is that, placed in the same conditions, he employs the same words as I and reacts in the same manner. But here is another person, who, although employing the word green, uses it under conditions where neither my neighbour nor I employ it, and I am able to declare that he has a definite defect in colour vision.

From this I understand clearly that if I were totally colourblind and had no sensation of colour—as I do become momentarily in a dazzling light, and as I am always in a very weak light—I would be able nevertheless to study the sensation of green and colour vision by the method of verbal responses.

If now I lost at a certain moment the capacity to experience sensations of colour, either as perceived or imagined, and at the same time the capacity to react specifically to different luminous stimuli, I would nevertheless preserve the idea—thanks to the verbal notations previously recorded in my mind—that at a previous time I had perceived green under the action of certain radiations.

Thus it is that the entire domain of psychological studies, considered as having to do with the phenomena of consciousness, is concerned in reality with particular forms of activity, of behaviour, of characteristic modes of reaction, principally verbal.

It is certain that for myself, whether I am concerned with physics, with chemistry or with psychology, everything is a conscious impression. But, among others, the word green or the word sensation has not necessarily a more subjective signification than the word cube or the word atom.[1] By methods of training which produce specific reactions to light stimuli of different radiations, as a substitute for the verbal reactions acquired in the course of social training, I am likewise able to study colour vision among animals. Perhaps they have conscious impressions, but I have no certainty of this; perhaps their impressions are qualitatively identical with mine, but that is not important. What is important is that certain stimuli arouse *specific reactions*, which appear and disappear under the same conditions.[2] The agreement in behaviour is sufficient, without it being necessary to invoke an agreement between mysterious processes which are omitted from the whole investigation.

I am able to follow the play of states of consciousness in myself; but as soon as I wish to express them, to secure a notation, I must utilize the verbal symbolism which I get from society; and the significance of this symbolism, transmitted from individual to individual, can only be founded on phenomena which are the material of common perception, upon objective phenomena. When a mother shows to her young child an animal or a man in pain, she will connect the word " suffering " to a mimicry consisting of the attitudes, gestures, actions and words which her child perceives at the same time as she does. When the child experiences suffering, he will know, by the correspondence of his own reactions with those which he had previously observed, that the word suffering then applies.

[1] We have already noticed that a deaf physicist, J. Sauveur, was one of the first to study musical audition.

[2] This idea is beginning to spread. Very rigorously set forth by Huxley in connection with animal psychology, and accepted by various biologists, it has been taken up by the sociologists, who are accustomed to observe human activities in their purely objective aspect—M. Halbwachs, for example. It has been clearly set forth by the surgeon Pierre Delbet in his work on *La Science et la Réalité* (1914) : " Certain psychologists are very much concerned to know whether the same causes produce the same sensations in all men. We designate sensations by adjectives which we apply to objects. When we say that a body is ' rouge,' that is intended to mean, in the language of the ignorant, that it causes a certain sensation. Is this sensation the same for all ? That is a question which is badly stated. It is an imaginary problem. The only important thing is that all men who speak French apply the term ' rouge ' to the same body in the same light."

As for purely subjective states, which cannot furnish any specific manifestation that may be an object of perception, the symbolism I would have to adopt would be useless if it did not have communicable significance. We may try to arouse inexpressible nuances by some sort of contagion, by means of musical expression, for example; but we cannot integrate these in a science. Science represents in effect a body of communicable experiences. Moreover, because of its essentially social character, it is not only unable to include what is unique and non-transmissable, but is not interested in whatever remains incapable of objective expression, or cannot become the object of collective experience or be the source of social interaction.

There is a science of behaviour, of activity, of the co-ordinated responses of organisms considered in their totality. This science constitutes psychology. It differs from physiology in that the latter is concerned with partial mechanisms, with limited systems of reaction.

There is a psychology of animals, which does not need to raise the question of consciousness that Descartes settled in the negative, a psychology of children, a psychology of the insane, a psychology of primitive man, as well as a psychology of adults belonging to our civilizations. In the last case the psychologist may himself be the object of investigation; but, in the other cases, he is not a matter of particular concern. There is no essential difference of method. There is merely greater facility for obtaining reactions since it is possible to use a verbal instrument which is richer and more flexible.

In the practice of research, the methods of objective registration of natural reactions do not allow us to follow such details of nervous reactions as are produced in the cerebral centres in the course of the associative processes. These reactions can, however, be objectified by verbal means. The possibilities of objectification are, however, far from being exhausted; as is shown by the recent discovery of the psycho-galvanic reaction, and as will be shown undoubtedly some day by utilizing procedures for registering action currents.

Among educated people the significance of such terms as image, idea and feeling has been learned by connecting them with common perceptual experiences. An image is an internal reaction following, for example, the hearing of a word. It may be developed into a written representation or into a verbal description which may lead to a written representation.

The reaction " image " may then be made explicit in a verbal expression, which will stop with the very word " image," or develop into a written representation or description. The introspection studied in this case, as in all others, consists of the learned verbal reaction. It represents a form of behaviour, of learned conduct. It does not introduce anything properly subjective, and is no more connected with the phenomena of consciousness as such than the movement of the hand pressing a telegraph key is connected with the hearing of the auditory signal to which a subject has been directed to react.[1]

However, the more flexible a method is, the more it is subject to numerous factors of variation, and the more it is under suspicion when we try to elicit general laws from particular facts, which is the aim of science. The significance of verbal reactions which the subject has learned to make use of often remains obscure and ambiguous.

[1] The idea that psychology is the science of behaviour [*comportement*], of conduct, has been set forth by Pierre Janet, on the basis of his pathological studies, and by myself on the basis of researches carried out in a parallel manner on lower animals and man, showing the common laws of memory. The "behaviorism" of Watson, on the contrary, has claimed —though with very little justification—to establish a new psychology eliminating what may be ascribed to consciousness. The " psychoreflexology " of Bechterew corresponds to a purely verbal effort in the direction of eliminating any language contaminated with conscious signification.

[In France Professor Piéron has given prominence to the definition of psychology as the science of comportment (*comportement*). In 1907 and 1908 he was the first to revive the use of this word, which is rarely found in French or English. In the translation, the word *comportment* has been changed to *behaviour*, which is the term in more general use. By doing so, it is possible that some advantage has been lost for the author's view which lays special emphasis on the organized, co-ordinated, integrated, and " global " character of the phenomena studied by psychology. *Comportment* seems to convey something of the idea of individualized activity which is not found in the more common word *behaviour*. It has also the advantage of distinguishing this form of behaviorism from more radical types.—TRANSLATOR.]

There are various degrees of precision and of assurance in the results of psychology, starting with those furnished by the conditioned reflexes of training, which are even then affected by a thousand disturbing influences difficult to eliminate, and continuing to those which must be regarded as introspective, expressing certain mental reactions. But there is no hiatus, no difference in nature.

In reality a contrast might be found between "auto-psychology" and general psychology. Following the natural tendency to report everything as if it happened to one's self, which causes the errors of "anthropomorphism," one often puts oneself in the place of animals or of children, of foreigners or of men of the middle ages, of savages or of the insane, and then pretends that the kinds of responses which one finds in oneself are valid also for them. If a particular group of experiences excites a disagreeable reaction in me, I have a tendency to think that this reaction is universal.

On the other hand the direct study of the behaviour of animals, of children (Piaget), of the insane (Janet, Blondel), and of primitive men (Lévy-Bruhl), shows more and more clearly that one is not able to pass at will from one group of organisms to another, and, though there may be common laws, other laws apply to any particular group. The comparative method at least is, therefore, necessary. The psychologist is not able to limit himself to the study of his own activities as he formerly tended to do, besides looking through the distorting prism of philosophical theories and preconceived systems.

Autopsychology is coming to be regarded as of less and less scientific value, although it has still its well recognized place in the literature. But, when regarded as a verbal notation, this autopsychology can still only claim to be concerned with behaviour, under pain of remaining otherwise as incomprehensible and impenetrable as consciousness. Popular psychology, like scientific psychology, is only a psychology of conduct.

Applying itself to studying the behaviour of all living beings, experimental psychology must be a comparative psychology, as Ribot very correctly stated; but the demands of practical applications lead more particularly to the study of man. Psychometry, as a general branch of anthropometry, permits the classing of individuals for practical purposes, such as their selection for professions. The laws of mental development furnish a basis for educational methodology. The laws which govern human choice, with its associative and affective factors and its susceptibility to suggestion, are utilized in the practice of advertising and selling. The laws of memory and of the mistakes of memory are the basis of the attempts towards a rational criticism of testimony in legal practice, etc.

The results attained by the scientific investigation of mental functions, which scarcely dates back half a century, are already numerous. They are being utilized now on a large scale. This sanction by practice is the best proof of the validity of psychological science and of its independence from philosophy.

Experimental psychology is often reproached for not solving the great problems such as that of mind and body. By making the same criticism of science in general it would be possible to proclaim its failure. But such a failure no more interferes with the continuous progress of physics, of chemistry and of physiology, than the failure often attributed to experimental psychology prevents it from continuing its fruitful work. It is evidently not the function of psychology to construct great explanatory theories which are incapable of verification. It can only hazard provisional hypotheses, submit them to the control of facts, and thus by research open new vistas. It has often undertaken to find in general organic phenomena the key to certain mental processes or to establish the social cause of complex psychological manifestations, but the extensions it is able to make depend upon verification and have only a provisional character.

Only philosophy, which undertakes to go beyond experience, is able to generalize or to oppose generalization, to affirm or to deny the irreducibility of the psychic.

PART ONE

THE REACTION PROCESSES AND THE FORMS OF BEHAVIOUR

CHAPTER I

THE CONCEPTION OF REACTION

WHEN a sudden change is produced in the surroundings of a living being, this change acts generally as a " stimulus " to the organism, that is to say, excites a response, which is a corresponding change carried over into its own activity, into the behaviour of the organism.

If I introduce a drop of acid into water containing Infusoria, the activity of these Infusoria changes in a certain manner. They will withdraw from the area where the change has been produced or they will go towards it, according to the nature and strength of the acid.

If I heat a culture broth containing bacteria, the microbes will become encysted and immobilized.

If I place, in a small quantity of blood in which leucocytes are circulating, some particles of starch, the white cells of the blood will absorb these particles after having broken them up into fragments and bathed them with dissolving juices.

The stimulated organism can displace itself, transform itself in relation to the stimulus or react to the stimulus, mechanically or chemically.

Besides these immediate reactions, the stimulus may bring about lasting modifications which will continue to manifest themselves in later behaviour.

I give some particles of carmine to Infusoria ; they will surround the particles and then throw them out again.

If I repeat this those which have tried to absorb the carmine will not do so again.

The first time the leucocytes are placed in the presence of certain bacteria, they will approach and surround them. When they encounter them again they will secrete bacteriolitic material.

Among these reactions, primitive and elementary as they appear—although their complexity is in reality extreme—arises the psychology which pictures in these obvious modifications of activity, the general behaviour of organisms.

At all levels organisms react to the same classes of stimuli ; they present the same general classes of reaction. That which affects the more highly evolved sensory apparatus of the higher animals, affects even the relatively undifferentiated protoplasm of unicellular organisms. Mechanical stimuli (vibrations in particular) and chemical stimuli, the radiations which they set up when they are absorbed, heat or photo-chemical activities, all affect Infusoria as well as man. No class of stimuli is known to act on man which does not act to some degree on the protozoa, and *vice versa.*

In the same class, for all organisms (although the extreme limits may fluctuate, in particular with the ultra-violet radiations), belong the stimuli of light and heat, and those which do not arouse any activity at all.

From the point of view of modes of reaction we always find certain displacements, certain activities, relatively complex, affecting the environment so as to modify it, and also certain auto-modifications of a stimulated organism.

Are these auto-modifications then in the realm of behaviour, in the realm of psychology ?

Following a toxic influence, when an animal immunizes itself, the modifications produced are not transferred in any apparent form into its total response ; they are consequently outside the realm that we are picturing. Only activities such as those which permit of an escape from a new toxic influence belong to this domain. Increased resistance to a snake-bite, after being bitten, is not a psychological reaction ; while subsequent flight from a snake, or learning the necessity of killing it, without letting it bite you, is.

Among the immunization phenomena in higher animals, however, there may be some reactions, which, taken on a different footing, belong to the study of behaviour ; such for example, would be the attraction of phagocytes, which represents a definite modification of activity in such truly individualized organisms, capable of relative independence, as are the white blood cells.

On the other hand there are some transition forms between incontestable reactional changes of behaviour and internal changes which belong only to physiology and physio-pathology.

In all cases where glandular reactions are produced we have to do with these transition forms.

Weeping constitutes a glandular reaction, which is linked not only with mimetic phenomena but with a whole behaviour situation in which tears are a very obvious element. Salivation from the point of view of desire for food is less directly observable, but forms part of a definite complex activity.

A gastric or intestinal secretion will in certain cases remain a sufficiently isolated manifestation to escape an observer of behaviour, but very often it will lead to active manifestations, it will condition certain conduct. The motor phenomena of the stomach or the intestines, closely corresponding to these secretions, belongs also, at least indirectly, to the psychological complex. Finally, an internal secretion will more often be a mode of reaction of great psychological importance through the direct influence which it exercises on the general conduct. The influence of adrenin, and particularly of the secretion from the thyroid, the testicle or the ovary, is considerable. The responses of the glands represent an integral and very important part of the psychological reaction—of the modification carried over from the stimulation to the conduct.

Emotion, for certain theorists, consists of its own mode

of reaction, implying essentially an auto-modification of the organism, under the form of " glandular behaviour."

Thus the reactional activity which the psychologist studies may, in part, be built up by modifications which are not directly and immediately apparent, but which reveal themselves by indirect manifestations or by subsequent effects. It is not only in the form of glandular modifications but in the form of nervous modifications that this implicit behaviour may be realized.

Some forms of reaction are preparatory to further modifications of behaviour, in particular the reactions which prepare to fix something in memory. Some imply inhibitions, at the time, of immediate manifestations and elaborations of different responses. This is the case with phenomena of thought excited by an external event, which imply particular conduct, the exact nature of which escapes direct observation quite as much as testicular or adrenal secretion. It is necessary that these phenomena should pass over into specific reactions, verbal nearly always, in order that they may be followed. They must be reconstructed on the basis of more remote modifications, as in attempts at the " divination " of thought.

Up to the present we have considered that behaviour was only made up of responses to stimuli, that it was essentially reactional.

The *stimulus-response* circuit which describes behaviour is sometimes viewed under the form of energy. The response would then consist in the utilization of energy brought by the stimulus. Light energy received by the eye would be transformed into muscular contraction and restored under mechanical form and heat to the environment.

But in general the energy received is many million times less than the energy given off in the reaction. The stimulus only releases a discharge of accumulated energy in the tissues (lipoids from the nerve cells, carbohydrates from the muscles, glycogen from the reserves in the liver, etc.). The energy of responses is furnished by the nourishment acquired and has to do with the general cycle of metabolism. But the organism uses in a continuous manner a part of this energy for uninterrupted functions or for periodical functions which do not appear to require special stimuli; and it uses in a discontinuous manner another part, for functions which require the action of a factor suitable to set them going, especially for processes of the relational activity of behaviour.

Moreover the stimuli capable of releasing responses are not necessarily external processes. There exists among multi-cellular organisms a general internal condition, the proper changes in which—often following a reaction to an external stimulus—are capable of acting in their turn as sources of stimulation. Thus it is that changes in the position of the limbs, movements of the stomach, etc., represent psychogenic excitations which arouse perceptive reactions; the products of digestion in the blood often cause an impression of euphoria; hallucinations, that is, sensations which arise in the absence of the appropriate external stimuli, are caused by the direct influence on the nerve elements of toxic substances introduced internally through the blood or the lymph which bathe them, etc.

Some processes, apparently continuous or with their own periodicity, may be kept up in the organism by this cycle of auto-stimulation in which each response constitutes the source of a fresh excitation.

In the phenomena of thought, prolonged for some time, it may well be that the mental reactions which succeed each other are each thus aroused by the preceding reaction.

Nevertheless it is doubtful, in the case of mental activity and of unified activity of organisms, whether automatism can be continued indefinitely. It seems that external stimuli are necessary, at least from time to time and perhaps continually, in order to maintain synthetic and unified behaviour.

In that inferior form of mental activity which constitutes the dream and in absent-minded behaviour, sensory stimuli intervene to some degree. Experiments show that stimuli during sleep arouse mental reactions, although unadapted.

Some animals, if external influences are largely removed (in silence, in darkness or when immobilized), fall into an hypnotic state, characterized by the loss of all activity.[1] Boris Sidis has obtained the same effect among young children.

There have also been described among human adults very similar phenomena, of unconquerable torpor and sleep occurring in individuals affected by cutaneous anæsthesia, deprived of auditory and light stimuli. Reference may be made to the celebrated but dubious case reported by Strümpell, and observations by Féron, Bregmann, Paris and Laforgue, etc.

Behaviour may thus appear actually to be constituted by a reactional activity excited by rapid changes in the environment.

[1] Among reptiles and amphibians the suppression of cutaneous excitations, by entirely anæsthetizing or removing the skin, is sufficient to produce a state of inactivity approaching almost to coma, with suppression also of respiratory movements, so that strong stimuli will not awaken the activity of the animals (experiments by Ozorio de Almeida and H. Piéron).

Chapter II

THE HEREDITARY FORMS OF BEHAVIOUR

REFLEXES AND AUTOMATISMS

CERTAIN divisions are often distinguished among the reactional processes. Tropisms, reflexes, instinctive acts and intelligent acts have been suggested. Tropisms, according to the conception of Loeb, consist of reactions of orientation towards an excitant, which result in making symmetrical a formerly asymmetrical stimulation. The mechanism provides for direct transmission of the energy of the excitant into motor discharge. A butterfly receives more light in the left eye ; the light energy is carried to the muscles of the wings on the other side ; these act more energetically until the consequent rotation places the animal face to face with the source of light ; and, from that moment, since the two sides of the body receive the same quantity of energy, rectilinear flight conducts the animal towards the light.

In reflexes the nervous system comes into play ; there is an activity of the organism, a *reaction*, while in the tropism the organism appears to have submitted passively. However, according to McDougall, this reflex reaction is not adaptive (" purposive "). Adaptation, the direction of responses towards ends, manifests itself with instinct. Bergson regards instinct as an intuitive reaction of some sort, a manifestation of the spontaneity of the *élan vital*, entirely different from intelligent activities.

The sharp distinctions made among the reactional processes, however, are the work of theorists. They do not express facts but are speculative conceptions. The word tropism may be reserved for certain categories of reaction implying an orientation response, which is static or dynamic, depending upon the relation to the source of excitation. But these reactions are characteristically reflex. They always imply the participation of the nervous system when that has been differentiated. (The labyrinthine reactions of man are regarded by Loeb as tropisms.) We know that there is never transformation of light energy, which is weak, into motor energy, which is of a totally different order of intensity. Instead there is a release by the excitant of a discharge of the proper amount of energy. This is true in tropisms as in all other reflexes.

May not the reflex be differentiated from other reactions in that it does not have the purposefulness of the others ? Although the reflexes are fixed in form, they generally have an evident function. A sudden noise sets up in the cat a reflex of the eyes which directs them towards the source of the sound, even when the cerebral cortex has been destroyed. On the other hand, even if harmful instincts are not common—for the species in which they are found disappear quickly—there are always sufficient examples to prevent adopting a differential criterion founded on purpose. There is the liking of certain mammals for deadly poisonous plants and the care taken by others for certain forms of parasites which are destructive of their colonies, etc.

With more reason the reflex may be contrasted with instinct as a partial reaction compared to a combined activity. Moreover, the division thus made corresponds to our need for classification. We quickly understand how all the transitions fall between the types corresponding to the rubrics, which are uniquely valuable as the headings of chapters.

We know of some reflexes which evidently imply a partial response without appreciable effect on the general behaviour. If we strike a sharp blow with the edge of the hand against the knee of a person who is seated, we notice that the leg will be extended forward suddenly as if to kick. This reaction is irresistible, but is limited to this movement which is quickly over. What a contrast with the complex activities of a cat satisfying the demands of her maternal instincts !

If we find narrowly limited reflex responses, we know also that when there is a decided increase in the intensity of stimuli this will produce a multiplication and spread of the reflexes. Certain stimuli excite many responses. If a drop of acid is placed on the skin of a decerebrate frog it will produce reflexes of the foot to remove the acid. If the foot is held the opposite foot will be brought into play. When the hand is placed in a vessel containing very hot or very cold water, it will produce vascular reactions of dilation or constriction, and movements to withdraw the hand which may be more or less restrained, but which are in the nature of reflexes, etc.

A pinch of the skin, if gradually increased, will cause a dilation of the pupil, an acceleration of the heart, flow of blood to the face, secretion of adrenalin and more or less general movements of defence. A cat deprived of its cerebral cortex when thus pinched will mew, claw awkwardly with its feet and make movements of defence in the appropriate direction.

All these reflexes may be considered as truly instinctive acts. Moreover, it is possible to increase the intensity of a stimulus so that it will pass over from a specific response into a general reaction involving the co-ordinated behaviour of the whole organism.

In the conduct of an individual the play of the reflexes holds an important place. The highest activity consists above all in maintaining control of this interplay of the reflexes.

The new-born child has all the equipment of reflex responses (sucking, grasping when the skin of the hand is stimulated, etc.). Walking is carried on by a mechanism which is mainly connected with the medulla. It corresponds to an automatic activity which is kept up like a circular reflex when released by a signal from a higher centre. The co-ordinated movements of the eyes are essentially reflex and yet they become a fixed habit only with the intervention of the appropriate stimuli. Whirl

c

around for a few moments and you will not be able to fixate an object without arousing nystagmatic reflexes originating in the labyrinth of the ear. In reading we ignore the pauses and jumps of the eye across the page although we utilize their automatic functioning.

The appropriate utilization of the reflex activities requires an integration, a control of these reactions. There is a re-enforcement or inhibition of partial responses through the unification of the total behaviour of the organism. The nervous mechanism starts specific responses, but the combined results alone are important for psychological study.[1]

The main fact is that the organism possesses inner systems of responses to certain categories of stimuli, which are variable in their form and in their complexity, in accordance with the nature and the intensity of the stimulus, and which are more or less grossly adapted. These systems of responses will be called, according to their degree of complication and extension, reflex or instinctive activities, without there being any essential difference between the reactional processes thus differently named.

The number and importance of these hereditary equipments is recognized for animals, especially for insects, but this is not generally true for human behaviour.

From the fact that the regulation developed for these processes is variable, it is concluded that we have to do only with a new form of reaction which is acquired by practice during the life of the individual. But it seems clear that the spatial reactions are more or less essentially congenital. These include movements of the eyes in following objects, accommodation and convergence varying according to distance, displacements of the head and the eyes to the side where a noise is heard, movement of the hand on the same side directed towards a region of the

---

[1] An attempt to set forth the actual effects on the physiological processes will be found in a book which I recently published, *Thought and the Brain* (in the International Library, uniform with the present work).

skin which has been stimulated (the latter occurs in infants without a brain or in a state of coma), etc.

These reflex activities call for psychological study to the extent that they are found integrated in the unified and co-ordinated behaviour of the organism.[1]

---

[1] It is supposed that the young child " learns " to walk ; in reality the child waits for the development of the automatic nervous apparatus for walking, which he will have to learn to master. " If each of the movements of our walking required thought," said Ch. Foix, " walking would be a gymnastic accomplishment which could not be acquired in thirty years, and the promenade of a hundred yards would require superhuman effort to direct and to will. Happily the automatisms are there, which the brain directs and co-ordinates somewhat after the manner of a master of industry." (" L'Automatisme médullaire," in *Questions neurologiques d'actualité,*" 1922, p. 402.)

CHAPTER III

INDIVIDUAL BEHAVIOUR AND THE
VARIABILITY OF RESPONSES

IF there exist in an organism certain mechanisms already prepared, which require only an effective stimulus in order to release them, it follows that in order to have a unified, individualized organism, there must be a co-ordination, an integration of these partial mechanisms. In the lower species of Metazoa, approaching a colony organization, which is perhaps the first multi-cellular form, the individualization is not complete. Some segments may show a relatively independent life. Among the Echinoderms various stages of individual unification may be observed. According to Uexküll, the sea-urchin may be regarded as a " republic of reflexes." Little by little the individual acquires, along with a large number of independent hereditary activities, the capacity of control, that is to say, the requirements of the synthetic behaviour of the organism are superimposed on the partial tendencies.

A form of behaviour intervenes[1] which may be called voluntary by utilizing the objective criterion of synthetic activity. If a reflex movement of withdrawal of the hand plunged in very hot water is produced, the reflex will occur normally in the course of a comatose state when the mental functions of co-ordination and of individualization of conduct are abolished. This reflex movement of withdrawal will be re-enforced and accelerated if previous sensory results, previous experiences, indicate that there is danger of a severe burn. The result is that the hand will remain a shorter time in the water. On the other hand the reflex will be hindered if another kind of factor inter-

---

[1] We shall later examine the problem of the significance of " voluntary " or " involuntary " as applied to the corresponding acts.

venes, such as anxiety occurring with grief, or a desire to manifest courage before assistants, etc.

Whenever the reaction is thus integrated in synthetic conduct it manifests itself as decidedly variable. Instead of being aroused by a single factor, by a definite stimulus, which provides the necessary and sufficient condition for it, the reaction seems to depend upon a multitude of present and past factors. The resultant may be positive or negative, it may hasten and re-enforce, or, on the contrary, retard, diminish or inhibit the response. In the presence of its normal stimulus, the reaction may not occur, but it may occur in turn in the absence even of this stimulus. In this last case there is more than the nervous mechanism under the familiar form of dynamogenesis and inhibition. A phenomenon of associative transfer is implied which has been studied by the Russian physiologist, Pavlov, and his students, under the name of conditional or conditioned reflex.[1] This transfer permits any ineffective stimulus to acquire the effectiveness of an appropriate natural stimulus, that is, to become exciting or inhibiting. Thus the flavour of a ripe pear will cause a salivary reflex which, by association with the appearance of the fruit, will give the visual perception of the pear, when it occurs alone, the power to make the mouth water.

The concept of the conditioned reflex is of first importance for the physiological theory of the nervous mechanism which lies at the basis of mental processes, or of the phenomena of behaviour studied by psychology and by sociology. The phenomena of associative transfer are the basis of all acquired tendencies and of all progress in conduct.

The variability of behaviour, which is adapted to the complex of circumstances of the moment and which profits by the acquisitions of experience, is the criterion

---

[1] The Russian word employed by Pavlov has been translated into French by the word " conditionnel " : the reflex is produced under a certain condition. In the English editions of his work, the word "conditioned " has been employed : the reflex is conditioned by a previous association.

which is called intelligence.   It stands in opposition to the
fixed character of hereditary automatisms transmitted by
instinct.

All possible transitions, however, appear to be found
between the completely unchangeable activity which
ceases to be suitably adapted as soon as there is the
slightest modification in the habitual environment and
the ordinary circumstances, and the adaptable conduct
which solves the most difficult and the most unexpected
problems.   All degrees are thus found in the variability
of behaviour and of the capacity for adaptation to new
circumstances.

The evidence for this is shown by the exact observations
and experiments made, without theoretical prepossessions,
among insects and among a large number of other
classes of animals.[1]

Just as fast as the integration of all the activities in
general behaviour becomes more complete the capacity
of the organism to improvize seems to be augmented.
This is because of the growing complexity of the factors
in conduct and because of our ignorance for the most part
of past influences which may intervene.   The   more
complete integration is correlated with the development
of the nerve centres of the anterior brain among verte-
brates and of the cortex among mammals.

The most complete integration, however, even with
man, does not include all the special mechanisms.   There
are limits to voluntary action.   Certain reactions cannot
be aroused in the absence of the effective stimulus   or
cannot be inhibited when the appropriate excitation
occurs.

It is impossible to inhibit the patellar reflex, which is of
spinal origin, and it can be voluntarily diminished
only by a previous intense contraction of the antagonistic
muscles.   On   the   other   hand   one   may   gradually

[1] Unhappily the observations of Fabre are not free from doctrinal
preoccupations, which have frequently distorted the facts.   On this
subject see E. Rabaud, *J. H. Fabre et la Science*, 1925 ; on the subject
of instinct, H. Piéron, " La psychologie zoologique," in the *Traité de
Psychologie*, by G. Dumas, Vol. II.

succeed in preventing the winking of the eye on the sudden approach of an object. Moreover this reflex may spontaneously disappear, by a progressive auto-inhibition when the excitation is repeated, in the entire absence of an intention to stop the winking.

It is possible to assist automatic processes involving muscles which are normally under voluntary control.[1] In all motor activity the complex acts are voluntary, but not the elementary processes which compose them. We do not know how to contract the muscles separately, nor do we know how voluntarily to contract our eye muscles or those of the vocal cords ; we do know how to make a gesture, to turn to the right or the left, to sing a note. We desire in our conduct to reach certain chosen results and the elementary reaction does not interest us. But if this reaction becomes interesting, it is often possible by practice, thanks to the mechanism of the conditioned reflex, voluntarily to produce some reactional processes which normally tend to escape integration.

There are individuals who can wink an eye at will, who can dilate their pupils, who accelerate or retard their hearts, who shed tears or vomit at will, who can contract the drum of their ears and let it snap back, who wag their ears or flex separately the third finger of their hands.

Certain of these actions are in reality voluntary only in so far as one knows how to bring about the effective stimulus. It is sufficient to look far away or very near to make the pupil vary, since its movements are combined with accommodation. By calling up memories of repugnant objects or sad occasions one may vomit or weep ; by holding the breath the heart may be retarded, or by making an intellectual effort it may be accelerated.

Furthermore, by repeated association of the idea of the act with the normal response excited by the effective stimulus, the recall of this idea may, ultimately, become a

---

[1] If one stands sidewise beside a wall and raises the arm near it above the head, with the back of the hand against the wall, pushing it with all one's force, as soon as the hand is released and allowed to fall, it falls automatically as if under a strange influence until horizontal and then descends slowly (Phenomenon of Kohnstamm).

sufficient stimulus. Then the act will occur under the same conditions as all other integrated acts in voluntary behaviour.

The limits of " voluntary " and of " involuntary " acts, that is to say, of synthetic behaviour susceptible of variation according to circumstances, and of isolated reaction processes, are therefore not very clearly distinguished. The same activities may belong to one domain or the other, depending upon the occasion. Such, for example, are the activities of expression and the imitative processes, which affect a large number of motor mechanisms and are not limited to the muscles of the face.[1] The limits of voluntary acts are modifiable, moreover, by education, or by training. The contraction of an isolated muscle, as well as a complex movement, can be learned if it becomes interesting, thanks to the play of inhibitions and re-enforcements which are progressively perfected according to the general law of the acquisition of habits. In order to become voluntary, to become integrated in the synthetic conduct of the organism, a reaction must be of concern to the total behaviour.

Among the organisms which we observe, and particularly in man, integration finally reaches insurmountable limits. Although extraordinary examples of strange powers may sometimes be cited, the organic processes definitely escape absorption by voluntary behaviour and are only indirectly influenced by mental functions.

[1] The reading of thought by the unconscious movements of the hand or of the oscillations of Chevreul's pendulum, which become more intense as one desires to restrain them, furnish very clear examples of these processes of involuntary expression.

Chapter IV

SOCIAL FORMS OF BEHAVIOUR

The conduct of animals includes an exploratory activity in the environment where they live, activities of seeking and seizing of food, of mating, of raising offspring, of protection and defence, finally mere exercise and play, especially among the young of the most highly-evolved species.

All of these forms of activity are found in man because of the influences regulating his conduct.

But man lives in society, and here at least the social influence manifests itself in two ways. On the one hand it transforms, it really socializes, even the most elementary biological behaviour; on the other, it arouses and sets going a series of new activities which are specifically social behaviour.

That social life profoundly modifies the forms of activity governed by congenital organic tendencies is quite apparent either from the rites of primitive peoples or the customs of the civilized.

The acquisition of food and eating are submitted to regulations which the collective group imposes on each of its members. The preliminaries to mating include severe requirements in all forms of civilization, and numerous prohibitions often bar the way to instinctive satisfactions. The constitution of the family, including the rearing of the children, reflects the organization of one or another social group. The acts of protection and defence also are not free, and play reveals the forms which the individual learns to practise in the social environment in which he is called upon to live.

Every man, in as much as he is a living being, will eat, make love, reproduce, protect himself and play, no matter whether he lives in one social environment or another or even if, under extraordinary circumstances, he grows up in isolation.   But, from the moment that he lives in a definite society, he will eat, make love, rear his children, defend himself and play only according to the traditional rules which are imposed by the collective group on his social behaviour.   He may likewise be called upon to abstain from eating for longer or shorter periods, and to restrain completely and permanently his sexual desires.

Furthermore, as a result of social life, new activities appear, corresponding to tendencies which, for certain people at least, have already inscribed themselves in the hereditary equipment of the individual, but which develop and acquire a definite form only under educational influence.

The fundamental category of social behaviour proper is what may be called co-operation.   Prior to man, it is found in groups of mammals or birds and in insect societies.   There exists, for example, a tendency towards assistance and reciprocal use which shows itself in various activities.   An individual is seen not only to protect itself but to protect another or to seek the protection of another ; it is seen not to only procure food for itself, but to give it to another to eat, or to demand its nourishment from another under accepted conventions.

In this co-operative conduct a special activity arises which is of considerable importance because of its effects on development, namely, that of providing reciprocal information.

Even among the lower animals one may see signs of peril or of plunder transmitted.[1]   By a simple process of associative transfer certain phenomena of emotional expression, of fear or of desire, become signs of the imminence of danger or of the presence of easy prey.   In the midst of socialized behaviour, these signs become integrated as a desirable means of assistance ; they are

---

[1] Von Frisch has carefully analysed the forms of such communications among bees. *Cf.* K. Von Frisch, *Sinnesphysiologie und Sprache der Bienen*, Berlin, 1924.

transformed, combined and supplemented. The collective experience refines and perfects the instrument of language, according to the needs and the demands for information.[1]

Speech, or verbal behaviour, has an extraordinarily important place in civilized societies. It provides men with a means of acting on all others, it furnishes a way to transmit traditions and rites, it aids both society and the individual himself in conserving the results of experience.

All conduct tends to be reflected in a verbal form, even when it is not exclusively of a verbal nature. Certain authors would like to see psychology limit itself to verbal behaviour. According to Pierre Janet, psychology proper may be said to have been born when "babbling to one's self" first appeared. With the crack of a whip society would drive the mind from the animal organism.[2]

If we permit on the side questions of definition and of pigeon-holing conduct, we must always underline the principal role played by speech and by logic. The latter is developed along with certain language forms in the Mediterranean civilizations we have inherited.

Verbal activity and logic are of social origin and are linked with a long collective evolution. Left to himself the child, who has perhaps hereditary predispositions which facilitate the acquisition of speech, does not speak. The example of the child born deaf, of the deaf-mute, is evidence of this. The forms of thought which are really logical do not arise from the mental constitution of the human organism as nature forms it. They require educational training.

Along with language behaviour, spoken and written,

---

[1] The spontaneous language of emotional expression likewise takes on conventional forms. There are smiles and masks for sorrow imposed by usage ; sometimes tears in the course of the ritual of weeping are a form of politeness.

[2] In reality the social influence introduces introspective conduct. It seeks to add to the course of the mental processes, beyond the reactions implied by their accomplishment, certain secondary reactions excited by them, which secondary reactions may be perceived and tend to take a verbal form. The psychology of the phenomena of thought properly utilizes these forms of verbal reaction and appeals to introspective behaviour which it develops and generalizes.

technical activities should have a place. From an early time man generally succeeded in providing himself with tools, which are only exceptionally used among animals. Man thus found among the objects and forces of nature certain aids which he has succeeded in utilizing to his profit.

In our civilizations, which have fallen heir to a slowly accumulated collective inheritance, these technical activities are numerous and varied and their importance is considerable. They are founded on the use of tools and of procedures for utilizing natural forces.

Connected both with logical verbal behaviour and with technical behaviour, scientific activity represents in its turn a form of essentially social conduct.

Side by side with science, in close connection with the affective and emotional life, a form of social activity which has played and which still plays a considerable role in human conduct, is religion.

Finally, art, including all the forms of æsthetic activity, presents again one of the most important aspects of social conduct. It is related mainly to play and to the sex tendencies, the social restraints of which bring about certain derivatives.

All these forms of activity, which belong to the realm of sociology in so far as the constitution and evolution of social groups have determined their appearance and their nature, are relevant to psychology in so far as they are realized in individual behaviour, and to experimental psychology in so far as the scientific study of the behaviour of particular individuals permits them to be approached.

PART TWO

AFFECTIVE REACTIONS AND THE ORIENTATION OF CONDUCT

Chapter I

THE ELEMENTARY AFFECTS

A TOTALLY different series of reactions follow the stimulus received according as we plunge a hand into warm or into very cold water. In an order which concerns, not the succession, but the growing complexity of the reflexes, there are first of all reflexes in the vaso-motor field, in the form of vaso-dilation in one case and of vaso-constriction in the other. Certain general reactions follow, either of acceptance of the stimulus with an appearance of satisfaction and an attitude of expansion or, on the contrary, reactions of defence with sudden withdrawal of the hand, grimaces and a contracting attitude. These two expressions are accompanied by various manifestations in the respiratory, circulatory, secretory domains, etc. Finally there are co-ordinated acts of verbal expression, extremely variable in form, showing recognition of the excitation and of its effects : " That is warm water, the contact with which is agreeable ; one likes to prolong it. Oh ! how icy this water is ; it gives you a shock ; it is painful ; I really do not envy anyone who puts his hand in it."

We have three orders of reactions which physiology shows correspond to three levels in the nervous system : reflex reactions which depend upon the bulbo-medullary or mesencephalic level, the affective reactions corresponding to the thalamo-striate level, and the perceptive reactions related to the cortical level.

37

Among all animals, including lower forms, after certain stimuli there will be seen positive reactions indicating desire, expansion, search for and pursuit of the excitant,[1] also negative reactions indicating aversion, withdrawal, flight. We see here the opposition of the fundamental affective reactions, the agreeable and the disagreeable.[2]

We are not speaking here of pleasure and pain which designate certain specially intense forms of affective reactions ; we shall return to them later. The terminology in the domain of affection is extraordinarily inexact and variable.

The agreeable and the disagreeable are designated by very different names : sensation, sentiment, emotion, affection. As all these words are used in other meanings, we shall say that these processes are elementary " affects," and we shall designate by " affect " the affective process in general. As a matter of distinction, the reflexes carry out well-defined partial responses to definite stimuli, while the affective processes register the total response of the organism, the direction of the general reaction and the attitudes of the individual being stimulated.

This direction may be positive : accepting or seeking ; or it may be negative : refusing or flight. Therefore, it is considered that there are two elementary affects and two only.

Certain stimuli, however, strictly speaking do not arouse either approach or avoidance and yet are efficacious, that is to say, they excite a general reaction, a response modifying conduct.

A cat strolls through a field ; it sees something move ; it stops and lies in wait, it approaches a little, explores, and, depending upon whether it perceives a bird or a dog,

[1] Evidently each of us knows by introspection the subjective aspect of pleasant or unpleasant impressions, but this subjective knowledge does not come into the objective determination of specific antagonistic reactions or into the understanding that we have of their nature and of their place.

[2] Corwin, with olfactory, auditory or cutaneous stimuli, has noted withdrawal as a natural response in man to the disagreeable, and expansion as a response to the agreeable, with relaxation if the excitation is prolonged or pursuit of the stimulus if it is withdrawn (*American Journal of Psychology*, 1921, p. 563).

it springs forward or scampers away. The initial reaction was preparatory; it corresponded to an affective process which governs an attitude of interest, of expectancy, and of exploration. The stimulation was not indifferent and ineffective. Whenever we hear a knock at our door the reaction of interest will be produced, which, as our expression will perhaps show, tends to be agreeable or disagreeable according to circumstances, depending mainly upon whether we are anticipating the visit of a friend or of a bore. In either case there will be a specific reaction of expectancy,[1] which will govern our attitude of exploration.

We have then three general categories of responses to an excitation, manifesting three affective processes: the process of interest with the reaction of attention and exploration, the process of the agreeable with a reaction of expansion and seeking, the process of the disagreeable with a reaction of retreat and of flight.

It is true that Wundt has conceived the elementary affectivity in a more complex form. He has designated six composite groups arranged under three pairs of opposites. It is a "three-dimension theory" of feeling, the higher affective states resulting from particular combinations of the fundamental elements. These elements would be: pleasure-unpleasure (*Lust-Unlust*), excitation inhibition, or depression, or calm (*Erregung-Hemmung* or *Beruhigung*), finally, tension-relaxation (*Spannung-Loesung*).

Wundt's followers, especially Meumann and Zoneff, endeavoured to demonstrate this theory of their master by experiment. They made use of the verbal expression of subjective impressions under prescribed introspective procedure, and of records of physiological expression taken for the pulse and the respiration. They have attached

---

[1] It has been found that the psycho-galvanic reaction accompanies the process of expectancy, showing a diminution of the resistance of the organism through which an electric current is passing. Wells has concluded from this that this reaction is not, as has been generally thought, a sign that an affective process has been set up (*British Journal of Psychology*, 1924, p. 300). On the contrary, it is a proof of the affective nature of the process of expectancy and of putting ourself on guard.

certain objective vascular and respiratory variations to the verbal reactions, called tension, relaxation, pleasure, displeasure, etc.

Below are given what would be the physiological characteristics for the six affective elements, arranged in antagonistic pairs with plus or minus variations of the frequency or amplitude of the pulse and of the respiration :

		Pleasure.	Dis-pleasure.	Excite-ment.	Inhibi-tion.	Tension.	Relaxa-tion.
Pulse	Amplitude ...	+	—	+	—	—	+
	Frequency ...	—	+	=	=	—	+
Respir-	Amplitude ...	—	—	+	+	+	+
ation	Frequency ...	+	—	+	—	—	+

But the experiments, when repeated outside the laboratory of Wundt, by Titchener in particular, have not given these magnificent results. It is certain that it is not possible to trace such definite physiological responses to specific complex states, nor to find, for these states, a formula constructed in terms of Wundt's three pairs.

It is desirable to try to describe the affects in terms of behaviour without the responses more or less expected by the experimenter. This is quite possible for the elements defined by Wundt. Excitement in the dynamic form, tension in the static form (muscular tone) represent a general increase in the activity of the muscles, of the organic functions, etc. ; while inhibition, calm, relaxation, represent a decrease in these activities.

But this opposition between levels of activity is a little forced. There is in reality one increasing series with variation in a single direction. It is somewhat artificial to consider the state of an individual, at the moment of an experience, as a neutral state like a temperature zero between cold and warm, Under the influence of certain stimuli, which release an affective reaction of interest, of expansion, or of retreat, in an organism presenting a certain physiological state, there will be produced an increase of activity. This may be purely static, as in expectancy, for example, or it may be dynamic. In other cases there will be produced a decrease of activity, which corresponds, however, to an increased activity of inhibition. But these variable results of the action of a stimulus are not fundamental processes and do not characterize definite feelings. There are active or passive joys as well as sorrows. The first effect of a stimulus, as it excites an interest in exploration and search or an effort to escape, is to raise the level of activity of the organism, either in a static or dynamic form.

The stimulus being of external origin, the behaviour is focalized in its direction. But it happens that the affective process is excited by an internal stimulus, of an associative and intellectual order or of a physiological order. The reactions, therefore, are of an associative nature and it is the mental activity, with its exterior reference reduced, that is exclusively affected. Some states of hope and expectancy, some states of satisfaction and euphoria, some states of anxiety and suspense, result from an idea coming to the mind, from a vascular modification, or from the action of chemical substances. By way of illustration we may cite the cerebral vaso-dilation and the penetration through the blood of the products of digestion that go with the feeling of well-being which follows a good dinner, the agreeable influence of alcohol, of hashish, etc. ; or, on the other hand, the diffusion of an excess of bile in the blood bringing on a feeling of discomfort.

The processes released by an internal stimulus have a diffuse character. They are not localized. They do not arouse orientation reactions.

Expectation, contentment, discomfort, correspond to processes—themselves localized—of attentive interest, agreeable or disagreeable.

But the difference between the two localization aspects of the processes becomes less when the external stimuli cause extremely intense effects, the diffusion and generalization of which masks their local origin. It is thus with the violent pains and pleasures. We employ the word pain (" physical " pain) to designate the disagreeable affective processes of great intensity excited by a stimulus. They set up reactions which are more vigorous, more

D

impelling, less easy to integrate in co-ordinated and considerate behaviour in which immediate responses are inhibited in order to give place to different responses requiring a more or less extended elaboration.

This pain is not connected with all categories of stimuli. Neither light nor sound excite the pain response directly. Occasionally pain is caused in these cases by a spasm of the iris or a violent contraction of the tensor muscles of the tympanum, and results then only from the reflex reactions started by the stimulus.

The most disagreeable odours and tastes will not cause pain even when they excite the defence reaction of nausea and vomiting.   It has been established that stimulation of the nerves of touch, of warm or of cold, whether agreeable or disagreeable, will never become painful.   But particular stimuli of the skin, pricking the skin, even lightly, will excite the lively and impelling reactions characteristic of pain.   Such stimuli are taken up by special nerves in the skin.   Pinching the skin very hard, some chemical stimuli (acids or alkalis), some temperature stimuli (sudden and intense cooling or heating of the skin) produce impelling pains, the reactions to which cannot be inhibited and which almost entirely escape integration in considerate conduct.   The reaction is carried over to the nervous network of the autonomic system.

Finally, these typical pains are caused by any violent stimulation of the covering of the organs (the periosteum, meninges, peritoneum, pleura, the nerve sheaths, etc.) by compression, shock, distension or inflammation ; by chemical irritation ; and by spasms of the muscles.[1] These pains are badly localized, diffuse, agonizing, and partaking of the character of emotion.

All of these penetrating pains are related to the stimulation of the system of nerves controlling the vital organs, the autonomic system, as are the cutaneous pains, with the exception of the pain from pricking the skin.

---

[1] Especially spasms of the smooth muscles of the sphincters, the intestinal musculature, etc., including pains from the intestines, liver, kidney, bladder, uterine spasms, etc.

The responses related to the system controlling the vegetative life, the coenæsthetic reactions to the covering of the organs and to the cutaneous covering, are reactions which are almost exclusively affective. They have no discriminative value, adapted specifically to the nature of the stimulus, but they tend to favour the continuation of certain influences of the environment, of certain conditions favourable to life, and on the other hand to withdraw the organism from certain noxious influences so as to protect it.[1]

Pleasures attaining emotional character, which are also connected with the excitation of the autonomic system, are not as varied as are the pains.

Eating or the exercise of the functions of elimination bring about pleasures, but these can scarcely be said to occur with great intensity. Only the sex orgasm, involving a peristaltic contraction of the smooth musculature, can be compared to the pain processes.

---

[1] When pains of internal origin cannot be related to a stimulus against which it is possible for the organism to defend itself, a state of restlessness is aroused among animals which causes them to modify their conditions of life, their feeding and their habitat. Among men an appeal to the sorcerer or the doctor generally precedes the change of conduct.

CHAPTER II

EMOTION AND THE ACTIVATING INFLUENCE OF
THE AFFECTIVE PROCESSES

PLEASURE and pain are emotional forms of the elementary
affects. Emotion is essentially an affective reaction of an
intense character.

There are emotions corresponding to the elementary
affects, the agreeable and the disagreeable, which result
from definite stimuli. Whenever these affects involve
diffuse internal stimulation the emotions are called joy
and sorrow, or moral pain.

But these are not the only forms of emotion. Corresponding to the elementary affect of interest there is the
" shock emotion," which is caused, for example, by a very
intense and brusque stimulus such as a violent and
unexpected noise. Corresponding to the elementary
reaction of retreat and defence there is the emotion of
fear ; and to that of expansion and pursuit, the emotion of
joy. Finally, there exists a general aggressive response
which is at the same time an activity of protection and
defence and an activity of expansion and pursuit ; this
emotion is called anger, and it participates in some way
in the two antagonistic forms of the elementary affects.

We have then the following table of correspondence :

Elementary Affects.					*Emotions.*
Interesting (Expectancy) ...	...	...	...	...	Shock
Agreeable (Expansion, Pursuit) ...	...	...	...	{ Joy
					⎧ Anger
Disagreeable (Retreat, Flight) ...	...	...	...	⎨ Fear
					⎩ Sorrow

The emotion of shock affords evidence of the specific
character of the emotions, since the attitude and the
reactional orientation remain identical with what occurs

44

in the course of the elementary affective process, except that their intensity of response is less. What characterizes shock is that the organic factors in the response are much more marked.

In connection with a relatively weak emotional shock, such as may be obtained in the laboratory, we find, besides some expressive manifestations of surprise, vascular reactions (peripheral vaso-constriction and cerebral vaso-dilatation), an increase of blood pressure, hyperactivity of the heart and of the respiratory muscles (quickened pulse and respiration rate), glandular reactions (manifesting themselves according to the nature of the gland involved and the intensity of the shock by an increased or diminished secretion) with which should be connected the so-called " psycho-galvanic " response,[1] and excitations or inhibitions of the tone and activity of the smooth muscles of the walls of the stomach and intestines or of the sphincters.

More violent emotional shocks, produced in very susceptible subjects, excite organic reactions strong enough to express themselves in evident responses. The inhibition of the heart brings about unconsciousness, cerebral vaso-constriction causes fainting or merely weakness of the limbs, relaxation of the sphincter of the bladder results in immediate urination, cramps occur with irresistible diarrhœa, feverish manifestations of shivering and chills are accompanied by horripilation (goose-flesh), etc.

Very marked organic reactions are shown also in joy,

[1] This reaction is shown by an increase in the intensity of an electric current passing through the body as it passes through the skin. It appears to be connected with the more active secretion of the sweat glands. It becomes more marked when the electrodes are placed on cutaneous regions which are rich in glands, like the palm of the hands and the soles of the feet. It seems to be a question of a progressively diminishing force of opposite electrical polarity. Dumas and Malloizel have observed in anger in a dog an increase of the salivary, gastric and kidney secretions ; they hold that the expression of the emotions is " polyglandular " (*Journal de Psychologie*, 1910, p. 62).

Other authors have noted in connection with anger in a dog, though after an alimentary secretion had been excited, an arrest of the gastric secretion (Bickel and Sasaki, 1905). The glandular effects may then be inverse, according to the particular case (individual differences, intensity of the emotion, preceding state, etc.).

sorrow, fear and anger, with certain differences depending upon the nature of the emotion. Sometimes a specific character is attributed to these either in their outward or their organic expression.

Purposive explanations have been given (by Darwin in particular) for all forms of emotional expression in man, in the same manner as has been done for all the organic modifications that constitute adaptive behaviour[1] in themselves to give it its specificity.

Emotion has also been characterized by the visceral and glandular components of the activity.[2] For Watson it is a form of hereditary reaction composed of fundamental modifications of the somatic mechanism in its totality, and particularly of the visceral and glandular systems, just as instinct is a form of hereditary reaction showing itself in the striated muscles.[3]

Thus emotion has been treated as a sort of visceral instinct. But ought it not to be admitted that every instinct has its muscular component and its own particular visceral component ? McDougall thinks that there are as many emotions as instincts, the emotion consisting of a specific affective process which accompanies the bringing into play of an adapted motor reaction. But it is by no means certain that such a large number of systems of specific visceral reactions can be found.[4] Cannon, who

[1] An excellent chapter by Dumas on the expression of emotions in the *Traité de Psychologie* (Vol. I, p. 606–690) well brings out the point of such problems.

[2] According to the James-Lange theory, emotion, in its subjective aspect, would be conditioned by the physiological reactions ; it would be the consciousness of these reactions. If one considered only the problems that are objectively and experimentally solvable, it could be shown that emotion was evidenced before the organic manifestations took place, and that these manifestations were not sufficient to provide for its special character. The conception of James and Lange has had an exaggerated success because of its paradoxical form ; but it has the merit of emphasizing the importance of organic reactions in emotions.

[3] Watson, *Psychology from the Standpoint of a Behaviorist*, 1919, p. 195.

There has not been agreement as to the definite and fixed physiological expression of the agreeable and disagreeable emotions. Brunswick, who has studied the contractions of the rectum, of the duodenum, and of the stomach in man by means of balloons introduced for making the records, has found many depressive effects in agreeable emotion and clearly stimulating effects in disagreeable (contact with

has directed his attention in particular to establishing the functions of the organic manifestations of emotion by experimenting on animals, has observed the similarity and almost the identity of the effects of fear, of anger, and of sharp pain.[1]

The significance of the emotional nature of a condition (an emotion), which would thus come to form a true unified state, would lie in its favouring muscular activity and the play of instinctive reactions. The heart beats more rapidly, the respiration is accelerated, the blood carries more fuel and oxygen to the muscles ; the stomach and the intestines stop for the most part their secretions, the muscles benefiting from this suppression of a concurrent activity ; this favourable distribution of the blood is to the advantage of the nervous and motor systems. Finally, a very characteristic phenomenon of emotion is the increase in blood sugar, in consequence of the secretion of adrenin, which stimulates the nervous system and shows also in the increase of blood pressure. In short, the emotion characterized above all by hyper-secretion from the adrenal glands, stimulating the activity of the organism and preparing it for defence and combat.

But the facts are far from demonstrating this general conception in a satisfactory fashion. There are phenomena of emotional glandular activity which are not always an arrest of secretion ; there are also excitations of the

a snake, firing of a revolver, etc.). He explains this by emotional compensation, a depressing emotion exercising an inverse action of stimulation as defence against the depression (*Journal of Comparative Psychology*, 1924, pp. 19 and 225). In summary, it may be said that the only certain experimental fact is that action exciting the viscera takes place with disagreeable stimuli. The conception of Allport that an agreeable stimulus has the effect of stimulating the sympathetic chain of ganglia, a disagreeable stimulus the cranio-sacral centres of the autonomic system (antagonistic to the first), remains purely theoretical.

[1] *Cf.* Cannon, *Bodily Changes in Pain, Hunger, Fear and Rage*, 1918. Cannon cites three observations of very different emotions showing identical manifestations, including vomiting, one with intense joy (Darwin), one with sorrow (Müller) and one with disgust (Burton). He studied these emotions especially in the cat, which from this point of view is the animal of choice. The hyper-glycæmia due to emotion, with its resultant glycosuria, has been studied in man. A dozen or fifteen students at Harvard, after participating in a hard football game, have shown sugar in the urine.

visceral musculature. Depending upon the intensity of the excitation, the reaction may predominantly affect the accelerator nerves of the heart or the nerves inhibiting it (the vagus nerves) even to the point of causing syncope. Can one be certain that loss of use of the limbs, trembling, sphincter relaxation, etc., which paralyse all defence, are truly purposeful ?[1]

There is a possible rearrangement of the facts in inverse order to the arrangement of Cannon, which may be stated as follows : it is not because there is a visceral reaction, chiefly of adrenal nature, that there results an increase of nervous motor activity in emotion ; but since emotional activity consists of the letting loose of an intense nervous activity, this discharge of activity spills over into the visceral sphere[2] and brings about stimulating or inhibiting effects, according to the part of the autonomic nervous system chiefly affected. The dominant effect would vary with individual susceptibility, circumstances, intensity of the discharge, etc.; just as in the case of pharmacological substances which produce stimulation or depression according to the dose administered.

In connection with the general trend of conduct which results from the qualitative nature of the affects acting on the individual, these affects also evoke a quantitative manifestation, which is indicated by their stimulatory effect on the activity of the organism.

Stimuli may provoke partial reflex responses, general responses which are already prepared (either through hereditary transmission or individual acquisition) and automatic responses. But a stimulus may also excite

[1] Sometimes a particular form of instinctive defence has been attached to facts called "shamming dead." In case of danger exceeding the capacity for resistance, inhibition and torpor might furnish the sole chance of escape. But while the utility of such reactions is admissible, it is not rational to include in this category such other reactions as trembling, goose-flesh, or diarrhœa.

[2] The paths of nervous reflexes are prepared by a sympathetic tuning of various incoming paths ; to act on such neurones as are not perfectly attuned, the incoming impulse has got to be stronger, and with this increase in strength its zone of diffusion increases. It is thus that Lapicque, in his general conception of the nervous system, explains the overflowing of emotion into visceral channels. (*Cf. Journal de Psychologie*, 1911, p. 1).

interest, an affective response, and thus bring about a general direction of the reactional attitudes. The latter demands a mobilization of organic energy.[1]

The nervous system discharges its reserves which are guided in the direction of appropriate reactions under the general influence of the mental functions.[2]

Furthermore, there is a certain organic overflow which, if it is moderate, may be favourable to the exercise of more intense muscular activity, but which produces incontestably harmful effects when it becomes considerable.

This organic overflow which is the sign of emotion, that is to say, of the emotional level in the intensity of the affective response, is much greater when the discharge cannot be made in the form of adapted reactions.

When flight is possible, when the danger permits escape, the overflow goes into efficient motor activity. But, if one is powerless, if it is necessary to remain motionless, exposed to the danger, if death is believed to be inevitable, it is the organic pathways which receive the uselessly liberated energy.[3] To the phenomena of exhaustion which follow strong emotions, may be attributed the serious disturbances due to the upsetting of the organic equilibrium which has followed excessive and chaotic excitations and inhibitions of the visceral and glandular system.[4]

Emotion should be viewed as a process of response, not

[1] From the point of view of the psychology of behaviour, there is an energy, X, of which the effects only are known. The physiological and nervous nature of this energy is a problem outside of psychology.

[2] When the mental functions are in abeyance, for example in the decerebrate cat having its thalamus intact, which was studied by Dusser de Barenne, the purely affective reactions are clumsy, badly adapted and little varied.

[3] For example, under the influence of the emotion provoked by a lumbar puncture, the excess of glucose in the blood, which indicates the reaction of organic overflow, is more marked among individuals who refrain more from gestures and spontaneous activities of defence. (*Cf.* Derrien and Piéron, *Journal de Psychologie*, June 15th, 1923, p. 533.)

[4] Accidents of exclusively emotional origin, of a nervous and mental order, as well as of a somatic order, were particularly numerous in the course of the War, and put very clearly in evidence this pathogenic influence of emotion (emotional syndrome described by Mairet and Piéron. *Cf. Annales médico-psychologiques*, 1917, Vol. 73, p. 183).

as a continuing state. The emotion of sorrow, for example, should not be confounded with melancholy sadness, which is above all a state of depression. If the sadness follows sorrow, it is a part of the effect of emotional exhaustion.[1]

In a given individual some phases of general activity may be greater and others less, certain individuals have a continuous hyper-activity, others a constant hypo-activity, others again a regular alternation of phases of excitation and phases of depression. The last condition becomes pathological when the opposition of the two phases is very marked.

In states of hyper-activity the association is frequently with an agreeable elementary affect, and the natural predisposition is for euphoria and emotions of joy or of anger. In states of hypo-activity the most habitual association is with the painful affect, and the predisposition is marked for reactions of sorrow and of fear. But there are some passive joys (Mignard), some euphorias accompanying a depressive state, and some active reactions of sorrow, some agitated melancholias.

The regulation of activity, which is in great part the business of the affective processes,[2] depends upon organic metabolism, upon glandular equilibrium. Depression of

---

[1] It is at the beginning of the emotional state that the characteristic effects appear. An Italian physician was charged with watching about 200 soldiers condemned to death. During the night preceding the execution, of which, according to the code, the watchman notified them, he observed that the announcement of approaching death accelerated the pulse very much. Then there was a slowing of the pulse, and, at each excitation, a noise, movement, etc., the emotional acceleration returned, but each time less marked ; finally the pressure was very low, the pulse slow and imperceptible. The phenomenon of exhaustion had been produced.

As for other phenomena, Gualino has noted the arrest of salivary secretion (dry mouth) and the excess of perspiration (cold sweat) : the release of urine and the paralysis of the lower limbs (*Rivista di Psicologia*, 1920, p. 42).

[2] In the absence of affective interest, sleep supervenes among animals. It is the normal reaction (" reaction of disinterest " of Claparède) which shows in the experiments on the conditioned reflex among dogs whenever the associated stimulus, which habitually announces nourishment, is not given, and when the expectancy of the animal is deceived (Pavlov). Weariness expresses an effort of reaction against the depression of disinterest.

activity, for example, never fails in the case of adrenal insufficiency. From this it follows that the phenomena of excitation or depression cannot be considered as specific affective processes and certainly not emotional processes.

Emotion, however, being an efficacious factor for excitation, it is sought after to counteract depression, as are also toxic agents like alcohol. The puncture among morphine addicts, by its painful excitation, is an element which often complicates the toxicomania for the person morbidly afraid of pain.

There is a mental defence[1] against the disagreeable affect which often accompanies depression. It seeks to stop this depression because in general the disagreeable affect then likewise ceases.

Restating the matter, we may say that excitation and depression represent quantitative levels of activity which must not be confounded with affective processes, however closely associated they may be with the latter or how generally dependent they may be upon them. Emotion represents a form of hyper-activity of the affective processes, freeing a large quantity of disposable energy. This overflows mainly in the sphere of the vegetative functions, and more largely when the motor reactions have less opportunity to be carried out.

[1] Boas regards this psychical defence as a reaction which no longer seeks to modify the harmful stimulus or to remove it, but to modify the organism, to render it, for example, insensible to the disagreeable action (inhibition, suppression). Certain animals when a limb is wounded and painful, gnaw it off ; the psychical defence acts as a mental autotomy. Boas thinks that he has found evidence of physiological reactions characteristic of this mode of defence (*La défense psychique*, 1924).

CHAPTER III

INSTINCTIVE ACTIVITIES

TENDENCIES AND NEEDS

BESIDES exciting an affective response through their excessive intensity, and their direct capacity to exert a disagreeable or agreeable influence, stimuli may acquire an affective value by association and transfer.

The approach of fire, which has previously caused a burn, will excite defence reactions and awaken fear.

Animals have been seen to flee from fire, of which they have an innate terror, without having any experience of being burned. Theoretically this might be regarded as an ancestral transfer transmitted by heredity, but the fact before us is the existence of a congenital capacity for affective reactions in the presence of one definite stimulus or another.

The sight of a mouse excites a very lively interest in a kitten which has not had any previous personal experience of that animal. It thus releases an activity of hunting and pursuit. The barking of a dog, heard for the first time, excites, on the contrary, an attitude of defence and the activity of flight.

These are called instincts of hunting and of flight, which thus manifest themselves. What is called " instinct " is the system of complex activity which shows itself, like a reflex response, on the first excitation, and which is found wholly prepared in the organism. It does not require individual acquisition or previous training.

A stimulus which thus excites the display of an instinct, possesses affective value proper ; it interests, it appears agreeable or disagreeable, it easily excites an emotion of joy, fear, or anger, and in this case frees energy which is discharged into the prepared pathways of instinctive activity, and which may also extend, in man and to a less extent in the higher animals, into the visceral and glandular sphere.

There are instincts in the form of definite activities, which are characteristic of certain species of animals. A certain mode of constructing a web intended to hold prey, for example, characterizes a given spider family.

The instinctive activities permit also a certain amount of adaptation to circumstances. The web of the spider will reproduce a certain pattern ; but, depending upon the points of support, it will be disposed quite differently. Instinct is an activity which is integrated with the general conduct of the animal. The more the mental functions are developed the more adaptive flexibility is manifested and the greater the variability. ın man the complication is such that sometimes the instincts are no longer noticed. However, the general directions of instinctive acts are still discernible in the midst of the variety of individual conduct.

The fact that the appearance of a young girl excites a lively interest and agreeable emotion in an adolescent youth and sets up in him the desire to show off and to please her is due to the release of an instinctive activity. It may be said that the stimulus arouses a tendency. This signifies that it has an exciting power and affective value in accord with an entire system of activity ready to be discharged.

A stimulus without any affective power, not arousing any tendency, any system of activity, will perhaps excite partial reflex responses, but it will remain ineffective from the point of view of conduct.

It belongs to the affective sphere of tendencies to condition the necessary incitement for all forms of activity ; to it belongs the regulation of behaviour.

Among the definite tendencies, certain of them are acquired through the individual phenomena of affective transfer. Social education implies the creation of a whole series of tendencies. The strongest tendencies, however, are those which are innate and correspond to the main categories of instincts.

There is not always agreement as to the exact inventory of the main systems of instinctive activity in man.[1] There exist, however, a certain number of instincts which are recognized by all. These correspond to the following general forms of behaviour :

The instinct of feeding, which is manifested in a narrowly specialized form in the new-born child nursing its mother, and which implies systems of quite different activity (grasping of prey, acts of eating, of drinking and of evacuation) ; the instinct of reproduction ; the so-called maternal instinct, the instinctive rearing of offspring ; and finally the gregarious instinct.

The tendencies corresponding to certain of these instincts are generally designated by a special name which indicates our social anxiety regarding the hierarchy of conduct, and which expresses in a measure the imperious character of the tendencies ; we say that they are needs. These include hunger, thirst, the need to urinate or to defecate, representing tendencies which manifest themselves with great force, imposing themselves upon the orientation of conduct.[2]

---

[1] According to McDougall there are thirteen principal instincts : the protection of offspring, fighting, curiosity, the seeking of food, disgust, flight, the herding instinct, sympathy, submission and docility, mating, acquisition, construction, and appeal ; there are besides some instincts of less importance, such as laughter (cf. McDougall, *An Outline of Psychology*, 1923). For Warren, the human instincts, twenty-six in number, arrange themselves in five categories : instincts of nutrition, of reproduction, of defence, of aggression and of social organization ; there also exist some instinctive tendencies, the realization of which is possible only through learned activities, including imitation, play, the predominant use of one hand, the relations with one's fellow-men, the realization of æsthetic expressions, and finally the acquisition of knowledge (curiosity). (*Cf.* H. C. Warren, *Human Psychology*, 2nd ed., 1922.)

[2] The need to breathe, connected with the increase of the carbonic acid in the blood to a certain amount, does not appear except under exceptional conditions ; the need to sleep may become impelling when it cannot be satisfied. (It is then conditioned by the appearance of hypnotoxic substances in the blood.) It occurs periodically, like hunger under the influence of spontaneous reactions : dryness of the eyes from the diminution of the lachrymal secretion, with an impression of sand in the eyes, closing of the eyelids, relaxation of accommodation, and a general diminution of muscular tone.

The force of the tendencies depends upon the instincts aroused, not alone upon the external stimuli which arouse them (sight of food, of an animal feeding, etc.), and also upon the internal stimulations. These latter may be sufficient in themselves to release the instinctive activity. The activity will include searching, if that is suitable, for the necessary external object, for example, water in the case of thirst.

It has been possible to determine the mechanism for releasing the instinct by internal stimulation, for putting the tendency in play, for evoking the need ; arousing the need to drink, for example, or thirst, the need to eat, hunger, etc.

Thirst is connected with the loss of water by the organism, especially in the blood, the saline concentration of which is increased (A. Mayer). Under the influence of this dehydration of the blood there is an arrest of the salivary secretion (perhaps by an inhibiting reflex). It is this dryness of the mouth and throat, as Cannon has shown, which causes the need, the tendency to drink. Thirst may also appear without dehydration when emotion produces dryness in the throat and inhibits the secretion of saliva. If the salivary secretion is re-established, in spite of the dehydration of the blood, by the injection of pilocarpine, as Pack did with a rabbit, the attempts to drink are diminished or suppressed.[1]

Hunger is aroused by the contractions of the empty stomach. On registering the stomach contractions of his collaborator, Washburn, Cannon states that every time the contractions were produced, the sensation of hunger was noted shortly afterwards. A cat whose stomach had been entirely removed (Carvallo and Pachon, 1895) no longer took nourishment spontaneously ; it had totally lost the sensation of hunger. The periodic return of the contractions of the stomach, through an acquired rhythm, correlates with the regular appearance of the sensation. In cases of prolonged starvation, hunger disappears completely (differing from thirst); as a result of the

[1] *American Journal of Physiology*, 1923, Vol. 65, p. 346.

suppression of stomachic activity, and the need for nourishment vanishes. This seems to be a fact which defies purposeful explanations.[1]

The need to urinate arouses a special activity of which the fundamental elements are the relaxing of the striated sphincter and the abdominal compression of the bladder. It is due to the action on the canal of the urethra of drops of urine which have passed the sphincter barrier (on account of extreme repletion or contraction of the bladder with partial relaxation of the smooth-muscle sphincter). Anæsthesia of the urethra suffices to cause the need to urinate to disappear, evacuations either taking place in a reflex manner or not at all.

The mechanism for the need of defecation is connected with rectal contractions and is also well known.

The release of sexual desires and of maternal love, which among the animals have only organic stimuli, is still far from being precisely understood.

It is known that internal secretions coming from a certain portion of the genital glands play a part in the release of sex activity. Among female mammals at the time of the discharge of the ovule there is a liberation of hormones periodically causing rut. The odorous secretions act as an external stimulus to excite desire in the males.

The genital hormones play a very considerable role in the behaviour of the organism. A whole series of activities and contest of tendencies is derived from the sex instinct. Thus old rats, slovenly and meek, after having received a testicle graft or submitted to a ligature of the *vas deferens* (Steinach) carefully made their toilets and showed themselves high spirited and courageous.

---

[1] Along with hunger, however, there are appetites directed towards certain substances and tastes which represent more specialized forms of instinct. One animal eats only flesh, another only plants, and the choice of food may be very limited. Some organic influences modify these tastes, these appetites. During the winter or in cold countries, the appetite for fats is much developed, while in the summer fat foods become distasteful. The female mosquito at the time of laying her eggs ceases to feed on flowers and goes in search of blood, which appears to be necessary for the formation of the eggs.

It has long been known that puberty shows in conduct by coquettish and assertive attitudes, by æsthetic pre-occupations, etc.

The body fluids have an extremely important place in affective regulation, but knowledge of their nature and the extent of their action is only beginning to be definite. There is very little information, for example, about the organic factors of the maternal instinct. The need to empty the mammary glands may explain in a certain measure how the cat comes to suckle her young; the satisfaction of quieting a local irritation may account in part for incubation by the hen; but there are other stimulations involved.

Rabaud has stated that the mother mouse during the period of gestation is very much interested in young mice and that this attraction increases to the end of the period. It is certainly not due to the action of the *corpus luteum*, but rather to a secretion from the ovaries. However, there is still in this connection almost complete ignorance.

The exact nature and the real factors of the gregarious instinct and of numerous social tendencies which depend upon it are at present no better understood.

E

THE COMPLEX PLAY OF SENTIMENTS AND TENDENCIES

THE regulation of mental activity and the orientation of thought are affective functions. The affective process intervenes constantly in all mental life, including the highest forms of intellectual activity. It acts on perception, on memory and also on reasoning. The dissociations from affectivity which we endeavour to bring about are for the most part arbitrary and conventional.

When it is necessary to describe the affective elements of thought they are regarded as sentiments, which are complexes thoroughly penetrated with intellectuality. The varieties of sentiments flexibly adapt themselves to innumerable situations. In the course of an individual's life the affectivity enriches itself by blending, refining and expanding in the play of sentiments and tendencies. It would be vain to wish to make an absolutely complete inventory, especially in our actual civilizations.

We have specific names for the attitudes and conduct which awaken in us reactions of inward recognition, and, in particular, which recall perceptive experiences that permit us to comprehend and understand the behaviour of other men. Thus we know the sentiments and attitudes of love, arrogance, triumph, contempt, hate, condescension, pity, etc. ; of humility, modesty, shame, timidity, respect, admiration, envy, gratitude, etc. ; of sympathy, cordiality, tenderness, affection, etc. ; of remorse, uneasiness, hope, satisfaction, astonishment, etc. ; of brotherhood, duty, obligation, prohibition, etc. ; of idealism, worship, ecstasy, etc. ; or of humour, the comic, the tragic, the pretty, the beautiful, of the sublime, etc.[1]

One may attempt to classify these sentiments and to group them from one point of view or another, but it is always quite arbitrary.

All forms of human activity which are not automatisms (in a considerable measure also the automatisms) and which are susceptible of release or arrest,[2] respond to whatever tendency expresses the stimulating influence of a complex affective process, of a sentiment, with differences in individual conduct according to the predominating sentiments and the degree of their preponderance.[3] Nevertheless, intellectual knowledge, the prevision of consequences of acts, will combine the perceptive anticipation of the end, the desire for the result, with the affective force which furnishes the motor impulsion for conduct.

How is this plurality of affective manifestations formed which is individualized in the sentiments ?   How are new tendencies created which do not appear in the congenital equipment of the individual ?

Thanks to the effect of agreeable and disagreeable experiences, tendencies for one or another fixed form of conduct may be created by the regular association of certain activities with the positive form of the elementary affect, and by an association of its absence, or of an inhibition of activities, with the disagreeable affect.   This is what takes place in the training of animals.   The training of children often occurs in the same manner through the influence of rewards and punishments.

There is another direct influence on activities, namely,

---

[1] No account is here taken of the impressions accompanying the play of thought which are also counted as sentiments, though of a somewhat different nature; the feelings of belief, of certainty, of doubt, of novelty, of familiarity, of absurdity, of probability, of mental difficulty or facility, of imminent recall, of comprehension, of strangeness, etc.

[2] The repetition of a favoured act realizes itself ; its habitua lassociation with a stimulus gives to the latter a capacity for release which may be sufficient, in the absence of inhibition, for the automatism to proceed.

[3] When a particular tendency has an excessive preponderance, causing, in the social life, a veritable upsetting of the equilibrium of conduct, it is designated by the term " passion."

the general tendency of imitation.[1] In the social environment there is a contagion of sentiments, of attitudes and of acts. This contagion plays an important role in spontaneous education by the environment. Thanks to it there develop activities leading to agreeable experiences. Community of accord in activities and sentiments produces satisfaction. These socially approved activities are, moreover, often of a form opposed to those which awake innate tendencies, such as are connected with defence and sex. The latter cause, as a consequence, disagreeable social experiences. This discord is shown, in one form, as disapproval.

Education, either spontaneous or directed, comes thus to repress certain natural tendencies. As a consequence it produces conflicts among the instincts, particularly between the sex instinct and the instinct of self-preservation or defence and certain acquired tendencies which impose respect for modesty or even the sacrifice of life.

Incomplete inhibition and " repression " may, in poorly-balanced organisms, bring about mental disorders and obsessions.[2] This repression reveals itself through the " complexes " which association experiments bring to light. These complexes are systems of images and ideas, in agreement with repressed tendencies, which awake these tendencies together with the preoccupations and orientations of conduct which they permit. The repression may reveal itself also by manifestations of disconnected activities, whenever the inhibiting control of social tendencies is relaxed, as in absent-mindedness, dreams, etc.

[1] Is imitation an innate tendency, a true instinct, or a manifestation of the gregarious instinct ? It is not shown in all cases among young babies as a truly general tendency. It appears relatively late. But some congenital tendencies manifest themselves at a relatively advanced stage of development. (See on this subject an excellent experimental and critical study by Guillaume, *L'imitation chez l'enfant*, 1925.)

[2] These results have been brought to light by Freud, who unfortunately has carried to an extreme the theoretical interpretations of results which are quite true. He has thus established a metaphysic of the unconscious where well-known demons contend against each other. One has social charge of censorship, while the other, representing the " libido," the affective force—exclusively sexual—strives to elude it, profiting by its distractions or cleverly masking it.

The educative influence does not really create sources of energy, but utilizes the strong forces of the instincts, directing and diverting them so as to oppose certain inner tendencies, to assure them a definite satisfaction only under forms compatible with social equilibrium. Imaginative satisfactions exist as safety valves for the repressed instincts. The novel and the theatre represent and develop these.   Art and mysticism are born in great part as derivatives from the sex and maternal instincts.

This derivation of higher social activities of a disinterested nature, is often called " sublimation." It shows itself in a growing sense of the hierarchy of values established by collective opinion.   Stanley Hall has shown that the combative instinct may find in rivalry a sublimated form especially useful to society.

It is difficult to determine precisely the origin of certain human tendencies, whether they are congenital or acquired, and how much the influence of education and the environment has on the whole affected the congenital equipment.

There are, for example, æsthetic tendencies and sentiments which exist among animals and which, it therefore appears, cannot be dissociated from sex interests. These include singing, dancing, and pluming themselves as preludes to mating.

Elementary forms of the impression of beauty, of æsthetic agreement, have been sought among adults and among young children. People have been asked to express their order of preferences for colours, forms, etc. It was thought that specifically beautiful stimuli might thus be defined. But the results have shown such a variability in preferences[1] that it is difficult to connect

---

[1] In regard to colours, Winch found among adults that white, yellow and black were placed, in order of preference, after blue, green and red ; but men preferred green to blue, red coming afterward, and the majority of the women preferred blue to green.   The order blue, green, red, violet, orange, yellow, white is most frequent among children of the white race (according to Garth, 1924). But (Michaels, 1924, and Winch, 1909) there are certain changes with age ; preference passes with age from red to blue. According to Martin (1921), violet, blue and red are

æsthetic pleasure with an isolated stimulus as such. Elementary forms of æsthetic pleasure are, moreover, quite rudimentary and often connected with simple processes of excitation (the stimulating effect of rhythms, of certain colours or of certain musical chords), although pleasure may be found also in depressive effects.[1]

The factors of variation are certainly numerous and active, but we may note a few of them :

Preceding excitations have a very large influence. For example, in a series of lights, the sight of white, which at the beginning was without interest, causes a lively satisfaction, a sort of relief after a succession of varied colours. Some impressions, disagreeable by themselves, augment the pleasure of an ensemble. The repetition of the same stimuli tends to dull their affective effect,[2] commonplace things, too often seen, lose their capacity for æsthetic effect, and too frequent impressions are wearisome.[3] Some more or less chance associations, give, by transfer, an agreeable value to excitations themselves ineffective.

preferred to yellow, to green, and to brown, the girls preferring red to blue, the boys blue to red.

These preferences, are, moreover, those of a majority of the subjects, but all possible cases are found. If a majority are also found always to prefer rectangles corresponding to the relation of " the golden mean " (that is to say, with sides in the relation of 3 to 5 or of 1 to 1·66), the individual variability is extreme and the dispersion of judgments considerable, as Thorndike noted (1917). The same remark is made by Valentine (1914) in regard to the comparison of notes of different pitch, or of different musical intervals.

[1] The exciting effect of red light has been studied and the rather depressing and calming effect of blue light ; although blue is often preferred to red. Musical airs have effects which are very extensively conveyed throughout the organism ; some of these effects which are depressing on the heart activity are clearly shown, with slow motives in a minor key, while the Toreador air from " Carmen "' or the " Marseillaise" have a marked tonic effect (Ida Hyde, *Journal of Experimental Psychology*, 1924, p. 213).

[2] Except for stimuli really noxious, the repetition of which only exaggerates their affective value, the return of the same impressions, agreeable or disagreeable, lessens their effects ; a person becomes adapted or accustomed to them. Some foods, the first taste of which was unpleasant, come to be tolerated, and a person cannot eat excellent dishes with the same pleasure when he sees them too often.

[3] This weariness explains the need for a continual change in the forms of art. A generation which has seen a type of painting repeated in thousands of examples is prepared to show a taste for an entirely different type, which thus takes on an affective value that has been lost by the first kind.

This follows the general law, which applies even to the relatively elementary functions of the nervous system, as we have indicated, and which assumes the form of what is called affective irradiation.

Affective irradiation constitutes an extremely efficacious generating mechanism for sentiments of æsthetic pleasure, particularly during the amorous euphoria accompanying puberty.[1] The contagion of impressions and the imitation of attitudes are on the other hand the principal means of æsthetic education, which forms the taste of each generation.

As in other social conduct, if the organic roots of æsthetic behaviour are found, the forms which this activity assumes in a given environment can evidently be understood only as a function of that environment. They cannot find their explanation in the individual constitution.

In the complex life of sentiments and tendencies in an adult, either primitive or civilized, the collective influences have a very great preponderance.

---

[1] This irradiation of persistent effects shows that we may speak of affective memory in the sense that the same perceptive experience will be renewed by the return of the excitations which had been associated with it. An impression, a sentiment, an emotion recurs under the same conditions. The discussions arise from verbal confusions. It has been asked whether there are affective " images." This has no meaning.

In literature with psychological leanings, numerous examples of the essential phenomenon of affective irradiation are to be found. Here is one, taken from Proust, and finely described : " Amongst other names of towns and villages of France, names which were only visible or audible, the name Tours, for example, seemed to be differently composed, not so much of immaterial images, as of venomous substances which acted immediately on my heart, making its beats quick and painful." (*Albertine disparue*, Vol. I, p. 200.)

PART THREE

PERCEPTIVE REACTIONS AND THE ACQUISITION OF EXPERIENCE

CHAPTER I

THE PRE-PERCEPTIVE ATTITUDE

ATTENTION AND SENSORY ACCOMMODATION

THE purely affective reaction of a lower organism or of a mammal deprived of its cerebral cortex, consists, in accordance with the nature of the affect, of defence or pursuit which is very poorly adapted to the excitation. But the flexible and varied conduct of the higher animals and of man shows a very precise adaptation to extraordinarily numerous excitations ; there is an enormous multiplicity of different acts. Reactions thus specifically adapted to definite objects are reactions of a perceptive nature.

The engineer of a locomotive connects with a red signal the action of stopping his engine. A red object comes into his field of vision, he abstains from acting, or on the contrary takes hold of his control and his brakes, observing whether what he perceives as a red object is or is not a signal to stop. But at the moment that the red stimulus has impressed itself upon the retina at any point whatever, there is produced a preparatory reaction. This fully resembles the reaction which precedes quite different perceptions, for example, while waiting for someone to come out of a room, the reaction when the door is seen to open.

This is a " pre-perceptive " reaction of expectancy and

exploration. It is still, for the most part, affective in nature, corresponding to shock and to interest. In its principal modalities it is reflex, but it completes itself in accordance with the first suggestions and becomes perceptive through an exploration which is already adapted to the nature of the excitant. If someone I am able to see only imperfectly comes out through the open door, I change my position, I go to meet him to see whether he is the person for whom I am waiting.

But the first reactional processes consist of elementary activities which are more common, those of attention and accommodation.

A light or dark spot thrown suddenly on the retina, to the right or left above or below, releases a motor reflex of fixation of the eye, assuring the formation of an image on the central fovea of the retina. This movement is accompanied by the convergence or divergence of the axes of the eyes of a sort which simultaneously forms an image on the foveas of the two eyes. Furthermore, accommodation, by changing the curvature of the crystalline lens, provides, in relation to the distance, a proper projection of the image, the clearness of which is thus assured.

The periphery of the retina functions only as an apparatus for pre-perception, a warning apparatus for releasing fixation reflexes. The central region alone permits discriminative perception of colours and forms.

When a sudden noise is heard, in place of this " fixation " behaviour, we have " listening." This also consists of a reflex reaction : the body is held motionless, breathing is arrested, there is a reflex accommodation of the tympanum and the head is turned in the direction of the sound.

In the presence of odours the " scenting " activity often occurs among mammals, for example, among dogs, in which case olfactory perceptions are of prime importance. In the presence of flavours the activity consists of " tasting " ; in the presence of cutaneous stimuli, " touching " and feeling of them. But, in the last case, the primitive reactions generally are control activities of an affective nature.   Exploration contributes at once to perceptive behaviour.   The spontaneous reaction to a sudden stimulation of the skin, tactile or thermal, is a movement of defence or retreat, a gesture of the hand in relation to the place touched in order to protect it. Exploration, as an instinctive activity belongs to the so-called higher senses, to functions essentially perceptive.

The reaction of interest and exploratory attention permits on one hand a phenomenon of general excitation which sets off its affective coefficient, and on the other hand a process of elective and directing excitation, with correlative inhibitions, which is properly called attention and which represents only a special form of a very general nervous mechanism.   If the voice of a singer in a choir is especially interesting, it is known that it will be heard, in the midst of all the others, almost as if it were alone ; the hearing of it will be re-enforced and that of the others weakened.   This represents an interest regulated by complex mental processes, but elementary sensory interest acts in a similar manner.   This sensory interest will give certain excitations a predominance over others.   It will bring out the suddenness, the intensity, the position or the unfamiliar character of the stimulus.   This always occurs before the perceptive recognition which permits specific reactions.

In the visual domain the inhibition of a stimulation through the predominance of another appears especially in the conflicts between the two eyes.   Our visual world, which we build up by rapid exploratory movements of the eye, is normally single, although the two retinal images are superimposable only to a very small extent.   The resulting image is built up as a mosaic composed of elements borrowed, when binocular vision is normal, from each of the partial images.

In looking through a stereoscope at two views which show characteristically different elements, it is possible to determine the contributions of each eye. These are known by the factors of predominance, which act without being known and without giving rise to an introspective reaction.[1]

Whenever two very similar excitations occur simultaneously, for example, two cutaneous excitations on neighbouring points, in the absence of a clear predominance there are produced two antagonistic reactions of attention. The result is a mutual inhibition overcoming the processes of re-enforcement, and the perception of each of the stimuli occurs less well.

In the case of continued or repeated stimulations the re-enforcement due to the attentive reaction manifests itself most clearly. Furthermore, the pre-perceptive activity permits a motor preparation which facilitates such later development of adaptive reactions as the perception will require. Sometimes this outlines the attitude which corresponds to a probable reaction, as the sudden noise of a motor-car horn, when one is crossing the street, incites running.

The reaction of sensory attention, besides the movements or attitudes of exploration, produces a muscular readiness which accelerates the motor response. Whenever the time is measured for making a reaction following a definite stimulus, visual or auditory, it is found that this " reaction-time " is accelerated when the subject is put on guard by a warning signal.

We shall later consider the characteristic processes of the phenomena of attention.

[1] With the impairment of vision in the right or the left half of the retinas, following an occipital injury affecting the visual centres (a hemianopic deficiency), a light stimulus which is perceived in the region of weakened vision, ceases to be perceived whenever another comes into the normal part of the field and awakens the characteristic inhibition by attentive interest. This is because the reaction of attention, with its inhibiting power, fails wholly or is too weak and unsteady in the region corresponding to the injured visual centre.

CHAPTER II

THE ELEMENTARY PERCEPTIVE REACTIONS

SENSATION AND ITS LAWS

PERCEPTIVE phenomena consist essentially in the adaptation of conduct to the nature of the excitation. The precision of this adaptation and consequently of perception is susceptible to variation.

The traditional psychology, even under the forms called " empirical," which are only a little less constructed by logic than are the " rational " forms, described an order of precision and of growing complexity in perception. According to this the primitive processes would consist of isolated " sensations," which would group themselves in systems and enrich themselves with ideas (acquired and innate) and with images borrowed from previous experiences, in order to achieve a notion of objects to which could be attributed a real external existence with spatial and temporal properties.

This point of view corresponds well with the method of logical construction of a mentally jointed puppet, which had been the procedure of classical psychology. Instead of observing how the social influences lead the human animal little by little to systems of thought and action which form for him a " spirituality," this spirituality was assumed at the beginning for man, as if it had descended from the sky to imprison itself for a brief time in an organism. The force of traditional theories is such that the power of facts can only slowly overthrow the artificial edifice which has been built with its attics in the basement.

In the phenomena of life we never see the elements precede the complex, the parts existing before the whole. The organism with its numerous functions is there from

69

the start.   It is by a continued progress that it diversifies
itself into parts having functional attributes which are
more specialized and more simple.

Conduct, and the perception which expresses its conformity to the diverse modalities of the environment, represent
in reality a primitive unity in the midst of complexity.

As soon as there is a sensory excitation, that is to say,
as soon as a stimulus arouses adapted responses,[1] these
responses well indicate the objectivity, the external reality
which corresponds to this excitation.   It is to a situation
that the organism adapts itself, the numerous properties
of which are translated into a large number of modes of
excitation.   It is to these various characteristics, which
are separated under a spatial or temporal form by an
effort of analysis, that the organism adjusts its conduct.

The examination of the perceptions of an animal or of
a child clearly shows the original existence of this
" syncretism," as it has been called, following Renan.

There are no sensations of brightness or colour, of
contact or of pressure with an infant at the outset ; there
are no individualized objects ; there is a garden-sun-dog.
From this mass, the garden, the dog and the sun will
become dissociated as independent realities.   Then the
bark and the shaggy head of the dog will be individualized.
The work of analysis, connected with social education and
conditioned by the symbolism of language, will extend to
the elements which are called sensations, that is to say, to
the simplest specialized responses which may be acquired
in relation to the environment.   These elements are more
or less conventional, as in the experimental methods of
psychology, or more or less socially natural.   Examples of
the latter are the reproduction of the pitch of a musical
note in a song, the reproduction in a painting of the
colour of a surface, etc.

[1] Anything may be called a sensory *stimulus* which excites in the
living substance a sufficiently rapid and reversible modification ; but
there is a sensory *excitation* properly speaking only when there is not
any response whatever, but a specific reaction adapted to a particular
stimulus.   Among quite low organisms there is action following sensory
stimuli, slightly varied affective reactions, but there are very few
adapted reactions, *i.e.*, perceptive reactions implying sensory excitation.

Sensation, however, does not completely exhaust the scientific effort of analysis, which seeks to isolate the elementary functions in the complex of normal reactions of the organism. Thanks to methods of training, specific reactions may be obtained to certain factors of variation in the sensations, factors which are called " properties " or " characteristics " of sensations.[1]

Reactions to quality are easily obtained ; for example, by producing a selective response to blue alone, or different responses to blue and to red. It is also easy to obtain reactions to intensity, with different responses, for example, to a loud and to a weak noise ; also to duration, as for a sound continuing for two or for ten seconds ; to an extent, as to a circle of light two or ten centimeters in diameter ; to localization, as to a flash of light coming from the front or the side, contact on the finger or on the back of the hand. With two sensations new properties become evident : an interval of time, spatial distance, order of succession, and relative position.

The elementary processes are thus made to function artificially, but not without difficulty, since the organic unity always continues. We shall have occasion to show this later. Thanks, however, to their relative isolation the relation of the two variables, the stimulation and the response, may be followed, and certain laws be thus obtained. These are the " laws of sensation." The nature of the processes and the mechanism of the reactions may also be determined.

We shall first examine the results which have to do with the factors of quality and intensity, and reserve until later the results which we classify under the categories of space and time.

[1] The dissociation of responses is obtained more easily by the method of the conditioned reflex than by that of training which implies general modifications of behaviour. By the latter method, furthermore, it is often difficult to obtain in apes specific reactions to elements dissociated from a complex (colour or form, for example), although the responses may be obtained quite well when the complex is preserved. Bierens de Haan has shown that a macacus which chooses correctly a red circle placed beside a blue triangle, is not able to do this if the red circle is beside a red triangle or a blue circle (*Biologisches Zentralblatt*, 1925, Vol. 45, p. 727).

A. Quality.

By varying the nature of the excitation it is determined how many specifically different reactions may be obtained for these qualitative variations.

At first it was determined what were the categories of excitations which could be perceived and it was stated that there were apparently perceptive modalities (which we prove subjectively in an analogous manner) corresponding to the excitations of certain regions of the body and certain receptor apparatus. The excitations of the eye were thus grouped together under the sense of sight, the excitations of the ears under the sense of hearing, the nasal excitations under the sense of smell, the excitations of the mouth and pharynx under the sense of taste, the excitations of the skin under the sense of touch. A finer analysis brought out certain discrepancies ; touch belongs also to the surface of the eye, the canal of the ear, and the mucous membrane of the nose, the tongue or the pharynx.

However, as soon as the receptor elements and their connections with the nerve fibres were determined, it was found that a common artificial excitation (electric, mechanical or chemical) of these elements or of these fibres produced the same categories of specific perceptive reactions as the excitations produced under natural conditions. From this originated the notion of the specific energy of the nerves, which was developed by the physiologist, J. Müller.

The analysis was pursued further. The sense of touch in its turn was divided. In the surface of the skin there are terminal nerve elements of different kinds which are essentially discontinuous receptors. To the apparatus of certain of these belongs the normal reception of mechanical excitations, to others the reception of temperature excitations with specially adapted receptors for cold and for warm.

In a single sense, which appears homogeneous, such as sight, hearing, taste or smell, qualitative distinctions are clearly found. The sense of taste includes four different qualities for which the receptors are distinct : sweet, salt, sour and bitter. An attempt has been made to reduce the extreme multiplicity of odours to a few categories of relatively homogeneous qualities. The sense of light is distinguished from the sense of colour. In the latter three or four fundamental qualities are found : red, green, blue and perhaps yellow. The pitch of tones, the timbre of sounds and noises are distinguished in audition. Finally instead of one apparently homogeneous quality there is found a capacity for perceiving qualitatively different variations of pitch in musical tone. From the observation that the absence of the perception of a group of high or low sounds coincided with a limited lesion of the nerve receptor in the cochlea of the inner ear, it has been concluded that there exists a specific receptor element for each perceptible tonal quality.

On the physiological side, if the connections of the nerve fibres from the neurones in the end-organs—which are associated with groups of reactional neurones in order to assure suitable reflexes—are followed to the cortical elements, which are themselves connected to the elements of association conditioning mental reactions, it is found that the specific character persists through the entire length of the afferent pathways and is still manifested at the level of the cerebral centres. In these centres hallucinations of perceptions without corresponding peripheral activities are produced by local excitations. The specific sensory character, from the physiological point of view, thus appears to be connected to the entire nerve circuit, the entire afferent-efferent system. From a psychological point of view it is correlated with a reactional systematization.

Let us consider, in the present state of our knowledge, the inventory of qualitative perceptions which are endowed with specific characters showing in the responses and adaptations of conduct.

The stimulations received by the retinas of the eyes are normally connected with radiations, the wave-lengths of

F

which vary on the average the distance of an octave (390 to 780 milli-microns). Among these we distinguish impressions of brightness, which are qualitatively homogeneous and vary only in intensity, and chromatic impressions. These latter are not all expressed in the verbal reactions provided by tradition. The number of these verbal reactions, these names for colours, varies, however, with the civilization of groups.

Four verbal reactions appear particularly necessary, but the need for qualitative specification leads to numerous notations in scales, tables and codes of colours. By progressively modifying the length of a wave of light it is found what variation is sufficient in order that the difference may be perceived, in order to have the possibility of a distinct reaction for the two stimuli. For example, one may be green and the other, let us say, a more yellowish green, or a more bluish green.

This sensibility for differences in colour[1] is greatest in the yellow and the blue-green regions of the spectrum, with lengths of wave from 585 to 495. It is least at the red and violet limits.

Normally about a hundred colour blends are distinguished in the spectrum.[2]

Light excitations, besides the chromatic quality which they show, are differentiated according to the region of the retina stimulated. This specific characteristic is indicated by the adaptation of the ocular reflexes. This quality is often called the "local sign." A normal individual will not confound an excitation above or below, to the right or left. But we should note that this quality may be lost

---

[1] A difference of blends of colours of 0·7 to 0·8 of a milli-micron is perceived in the regions of maximal sensibility ; at 530 it requires nearly 2 milli-microns, beyond 450 and of 635, it requires more than 2.

[2] Certain people distinguish more than 140, others only 60 ; these are the normal variations. About 8 in 100 men, the proportion being less for women, show anomalies, generally hereditary, in colour vision ; cases of colour-blindness. Complete colour-blindness occurs rarely ; it resembles that which characterizes the extreme periphery of the retina or vision in very feeble light, night vision. Generally there is a deficiency in red or green vision (Daltonism), the yellow and blue only being correctly perceived ; at times the blue-yellow vision is affected. A few cases are known where the colour-blindness is limited to one eye.

or at least much confused when the elementary processes of spatial adaptation are defective. (See the later discussion of spatial perceptions.)

Concerning the reception of auditory impressions, the natural excitant, re-enforced by the sensory apparatus of the middle ear, consists of mechanical vibrations of the surrounding air. The frequencies cover about 10 octaves, between 16 and 16,000 vibrations per second. There are perceptions without tonal character, the noises, and others showing a quality which varies with the frequency of the vibrations, known as pitch.

The sensitivity for differences of frequency of vibration varies greatly among individuals.[1] Certain people distinguish variations of the order of a third of a vibration per second. The discrimination is not alike throughout the scale. It is greatest within the register of the human voice (between about 160 and 2,000 vibrations per second) or at least towards the upper limit of this register.[2]

One relationship of sounds is found to be connected with frequency in a geometrical progression with a base of 2, It was translated by the community of verbal reactions into musical notation, which is to-day handed down to us by collective tradition. All perceptions corresponding to sounds having 1, 2, 4, 8 times the number 64 vibrations are indicated as perceptions of " c."

But the c's in the scale of octaves are distinguished by special symbols, C having 64, c 128, and c[1] 256 v.d.[3]

[1] Seashore's results indicate that among 167 children from 6 to 15 years of age, 20 distinguished from 1 to 2 vibrations, 63 from 3 to 5, 48 from 6 to 10, 22 from 12 to 30, and 14 succeeded in discriminating only a difference of more than 30 vibrations.

[2] If relative differences are considered, as in musical notation where the " comma " represents a relation of 80 to 81, or of 1 vibration to 80 (5 to 400), it should be noted that the differential sensitivity is not constant. In the optimal region the threshold corresponds sensibly to the same absolute difference, or increases much less rapidly than the frequency ; after that it increases much more rapidly than the frequency.

[3] There is no agreement as to the true quality of pitch. For certain people, the position of the note in the octave is irreducible, while it is by the timbre, the brightness and the volume that the absolute position of the octave is perceived. For others it is the position of the octave which corresponds to the irreducible perception of height, the periodical relationship of notes bringing about the existence of the common overtones, so that the relationship would disappear for entirely pure tones.

The requirements of music have thus given birth to a system of reactions, to a form of verbal notation flexible enough to provide easily transmissible results concerning tonal perceptions and their specific excitations.

Musical sounds and noises possess other specific qualities, designated under the term " timbre." These tend to be separated into two components, the *brightness* and the *volume* of the sounds. This quality of timbre is translated by distinct and adapted reactions to the noises produced by the fall of different objects or to the sounds of the same apparent pitch produced by different instruments, the piano, the flute, the violin, etc.

Still another quality of auditory perceptions has been named. It is called " vocal quality," and is the third component of timbre (noises in *a*, in *o*, in *u*, in *i*, etc.) ; the vowels, in their vocal sounds, would thus be distinguished by their timbre, in accordance with this specific characteristic.[1]

The system of odours is far from having a satisfactory group of notations. Certain olfactory excitations are reacted to by the names of the objects which start the excitations. We speak of rose odour or of violet, as we speak also of rose colour or violet, orange and salmon. If we are forced to make a systematic grouping, which is still far from being possible, we distinguish families of odours as ethereal, aromatic, resinous, ambrosial, alliaceous, empyreumatic, caprylic, repulsive and nauseous. The last-named arouse modes of affective and reflex action. But there are always complexes which are very difficult to separate and the really elementary excitations are poorly understood. The odours proper are to be distinguished from the tactile or painful excitations of the mucous membrane of the nose, such as those from the

---

[1] In general a vowel is characterized as a particular complex of tonal impressions ; noises would be groups which are too complex to permit an evident perception of tone. There is, in sounds heard, a variable " purity " corresponding to greater or less distinctness of the tonal perception to the " tonal threshold," which is comparable to the saturation of colour, or the " purity " of colour.

fumes of ammonia which excites a pungent perception and causes tears.[1]

Tastes show four distinct qualities, sweet, salt, bitter and sour ; but these qualities combine in various complexes and are associated with olfactory, thermal, tactile and other impressions.

Cutaneous sensitivity includes touch proper, the prick sense, the sense of warm, the sense of cold, each with one quality connected with the nature of the excitant ; but possessing also a specific local character, related to the point of the skin stimulated, and including a reaction adapted to the place of excitation.

The inventory of specific perceptive reactions is not limited, however, to the sensory qualities thus grouped.

Besides the affective organic sensitivity, agreeable or disagreeable impressions coming from the organs, or from their coverings (including the skin) and from certain regions of the body, particularly the mucous membranes (which are a simple consequence of organic functioning, of irritation or of injury, etc.) there are internal receptive excitations bringing about specific reactions.[2]

The subcutaneous connective tissue, the muscles, the bones, the articular membranes, etc., are sensitive to mechanical stimuli, shocks and pressures. They furnish tactile perceptions which are difficult to distinguish from those which are connected with stimulation of the skin.[3]

Movements are a very important source of specific excitations. A perception of the intensity of muscular contractions may be isolated. This may be felt, for example, if one contracts the biceps while holding the fore-

[1] André Mayer connects with a special sense, which he calls " drimyosmic," the irritating excitations of the respiratory passages, which cause reflexes of defence, particularly the arrest of respiration.

[2] The impressions called " protopathic " by Head excite affective reactions, the " epicritic " impressions permit discrimination and are specific perceptive reactions.

[3] There are sensations of deep pressure revealed when the skin has been anæsthetized. Mechanical vibrations are especially well perceived through the intermediary of the bones, by reason of the selective transmission along the solid matter, and a summation by the excitation of multiple nerve termini in the periosteum. To the bones, therefore, has been incorrectly attributed a specific vibratory sense.

arm rigid. There is a perception of a pull on the tendons, as when too heavy a weight, while being lifted with the forearm, causes a gradual bending of that part of the arm. Finally there is the perception of the displacement of the joints, which manifests itself very clearly when we passively allow an arm to be raised. The origin of this perception is partly in the nerve endings in the joints, but it principally depends upon impressions of the sliding of the skin.

Displacements of the body in space are perceived by a mechanism which brings in a specific receptor apparatus in the inner ear (semi-circular canals, utricle and sacculus) ; but this excites only reflex reactions and it is only the perception of these reactions which brings about the full adjustment of behaviour and the mental responses.[1] We shall return to this discussion in connection with spatial perceptions.

There are certain other stimuli and specific reactions which have led to the belief in the existence of still more numerous elementary qualities, but the possibility of analysis, of dissociation, shows that they are complex, a kind of primitive form of perception. Our alimentary impressions, for example, include at times odours, flavours, or tactile results (smoothness and roughness) ; our perceptions of oiliness, viscosity, or stickiness, of gloss and of wrinkles, and our perceptions of form, imply results of pressure, of warm or cold, sometimes of pricking, or of the stretching of the skin, with the intervention of many distinct local impressions, and also " kinæsthetic " impressions which result from motor reactions of pre-perceptive exploration.

B.   Intensity.

Every sensory impression may be greater or less. A light excitation may be more or less bright, that is to say,

---

[1] This has to do with impressions called " proprioceptive " because their origin is found in the activity of the organism itself. Those which are due to excitations arising in the interior of the body are called " interoceptive " (in the stomach or the intestine, for example) ; light, olfactory, tactile and similar stimuli produce impressions which are " exteroceptive " (Sherrington).

more or less intense. Furthermore, if this excitation has a definite chromatic quality, the " chroma " itself may be greater or less, it has different degrees of " saturation," that is to say, of chromatic intensity, extending from a grey of the same brightness to a very vivid colour.

The researches of Koenig and Brodhun made it possible to count about 750 degrees of brightness which could be discriminated. These variations ran from the feeblest impression on the retina, corresponding to a brightness of the order of a millionth of a milli-Lambert, to the strongest accompanied by a bearable pain. This is furnished by the sun at mid-day, representing about 500,000 Lamberts. It cannot be viewed without endangering the integrity of the retina.

The degrees of perceptible saturation depend upon the blend and the brightness. Under optimal conditions they may reach as many as 150.[1]

In regard to audition, there has been little study of the intensity of tonal quality, of pure one, which is confused in the complex notion of timbre. However, the probable number of degrees of perceptible intensity between the weakest audible tone (corresponding to a pressure of a little more than a five-hundredth of a dyne per square centimetre), and the most intense, which becomes painful to hear (about 10,000 dynes per square centimetre), has been determined for an optimal tonal pitch (about 2,000 v.d.) and for the other discernible tones, the number of which has also been determined.[2] The rough integration yielded, according to Fletcher and Wegel, about 300,000 distinct perceptions from merely the intensity-pitch combinations. If the qualities of timbre were included, the

---

[1] The combination of the degrees of perceptible brightness with the average number of spectral blends distinguishable (about 20, less with greater brightness than with medium, almost none with the very weak) and with the average number of degrees of saturation (about 25) gives a number of distinct elementary visual perceptions around 750,000. If the local signs were included, the number would be of the order of tens of millions.

[2] According to the researches of Luft, M. Meyer, and Preyer about 11,000 tones may be distinguished, the most favourable octave (512–1024 v.d.) furnishing 1460.

number of elementary perceptions heard would be extra-ordinarily increased.[1]

The registers of intensities are much less rich for the other categories of sensory impressions.

How is the variation in the intensity of an excitation discovered ?

Let us increase the objective intensity of a stimulus, for example, by letting down on the skin of a finger pins held in equilibrium on their points. For a weight of a milligram any reaction may be recorded by repeating the excitation a hundred times. Let us admit that for a weight of five milligrams, 25 times in 100 a contact will be acknowledged ; for a weight of six milligrams, perception will occur 50 times in 100 ; for a weight of seven milligrams, 75 times in 100 ; and for a weight of eight milligrams, 99 times in 100. It is convenient to call the absolute threshold of the sensation the value of the excitation giving 75 per cent. (or, according to some authors, 50 per cent.) positive reactions.[2]

Let us now use our liminal stimulus of seven milligrams and produce in the subject no longer a reaction acknow-ledging contact, but one acknowledging a more intense contact, a stronger pressure. We shall find that, in order to have 75 per cent. of the reactions positive, it will require a weight of 12 milligrams, which is an increase of five-sevenths of our first excitation. Let us continue, starting with a stimulus of 12, and so on. We will thus determine the number of distinct steps of the tactile perception of

---

[1] For volume, Rich distinguished about 220 to 230 perceptible steps, but the variations of volume are quite closely connected with pitch.

[2] The variability of internal conditions really permits a numerical value to be obtained only by a statistical method. Below the numerical value characterizing the threshold, it is possible to obtain perceptive responses, or at least pre-perceptive (reactions of adaptation produced before discriminative reactions). The Müller-Lyer illusion may be produced by adding lines which are not perceived (Jastrow). There also exist systematic variations of the threshold due to preparatory actions (orientation of attention). In particular the threshold is always lower when one proceeds by the descending method, starting with stimuli above the limit, than when one employs the ascending method, starting with stimuli below the limit. The mechanism of this pheno-menon, which belongs to physiology (for example to the electric excitation of the nerves) is not known.

intensity, establishing each time the value for a step. For the first step of this " differential threshold " the absolute value was 5 milligrams in the first experiment, the relative value five-sevenths, or 0.714.

What is the relative value of the differential threshold when different levels are studied ? According to " Weber's Law " this relative value remains constant. With an intensity of 7 centigrams or of 7 decigrams, I will have to increase my weight by five-sevenths, bringing it to 12 centigrams or 12 decigrams, in order to perceive a more intense pressure (or to descend from 12 to 7 in order to obtain the reaction of " less intense ").

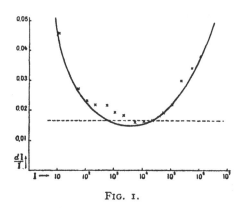

FIG. I.

Showing graphically on a logarithmic scale, the variation of the differential fraction which is just perceptible, when the intensity of light is increased.

(Experiments of Koenig and Brodhun in which the empirical values are indicated by crosses. The horizontal dotted line corresponds to a constant differential fraction (Weber's Law).)

In reality Weber's Law only holds very roughly. It is approximately valid for medium intensities of excitations, for the most usual intensities. For these its practical value is undeniable. But for weak and strong intensities the value of the differential fraction, i.e., of the relative threshold, is found to increase. (See Fig. I.) A complex law expresses the relation of this fraction to the absolute intensity.

If the intensity of the perceived excitation is considered to increase by an equal amount for each step of just noticeable differences, the relation of this increase in intensity in connection with the law of differential thresholds may be shown by a graph. Weber's Law being accepted, this intensity increases proportionally to the logarithm of the intensity of the stimulus (Fechner's Law). According to the real law, the relation of the curve of increase is more complex (see Fig. 2). Different mathematical formulæ have been proposed to express this law, one of them being by the Norwegian psychologist, Schjelderup.

On these " psychophysical " laws[1] an entire system of metaphysics has been constructed, the validity of which

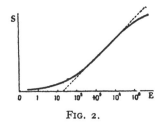

FIG. 2.

Showing graphically, on a logarithmic scale, the increase of sensation in relation to the intensities of the excitation.

(According to the measurements of the differential sensibility of light made by Koenig and Brodhun). The oblique straight line corresponds to Fechner's Law. It agrees in the medium intensities with the empirical curve of the S form.

has been contested because the phenomena of consciousness do not submit to a quantitative arithmetic like that which utilizes scale-units based on the intensity of sensation in the theory of Fechner. The metaphysics is, however, independent of the laws and the value of these is entirely objective. When it is necessary to classify objects according to the intensity of the excitation which

[1] The " Psychophysics " of Fechner claimed to establish a direct relation between the conscious process and the physical stimulus ; but the characteristic relations of the so-called " psychophysical " laws appear in the form of a transformation of the external stimulus into a biological phenomenon.

they exert, it is found that equally distant intervals occur for intensities of stimulus arranged in a geometrical progression. This is what the first astronomers did when they arranged the stars in order of brightness, by "magnitudes."[1] It is what any person does when he classifies greys. It is known, and this is a practically important idea, that if it is desired, in a design or in a picture, to use a middle grey, between white and black, and one which will really appear to be halfway between, an objectively middle value will fail to give the result. Conforming to the law of the increase of intensities, a middle grey will correspond to about one-fifth white and four-fifths black.[2]

We find also in purely physiological reactions (negative variation showing the intensity of the response of the sensory nerve) objectively measurable magnitudes which furnish a verification of the law. In particular the amount of contraction of the pupil exposed to lights of increasing intensity is found to increase according to the same law as the perception of light intensity deduced from the mode of variation of the differential fraction. It is exactly the same for the amount of negative variation of the optic nerve of a frog, when its eye is submitted to increasing brightnesses.[3]

The number of increases of intensity of sensation is very unequal, depending upon the nature of the sensation. On one hand, as we have already indicated, it is a function

[1] From the first to the sixth magnitude, the brightnesses do not run from 6 to 1, but from 100 to 1, which implies a geometrical progression with a base of 2·5. For a given factor (weights, for example), if the difference is known between the objective scales (determined by a balance) and the perceptive scales, there is a tendency to make a correction. In such cases the classification of magnitudes represents in general a compromise between the natural classification and the corrected classification.

[2] In his book, *Les Reproductions photomécaniques polychromes* (*Encyclopédie scientifique*, Doin), L. P. Clerc remarks that, if to 40% of a grey composed of 70% black, is added 60% black, the result appears to be about 40% ; while, if the same proportion of black is added to pure white, the result apparently will be only 20% ; and that this is due to the law of Fechner, which has direct practical importance (p. 45–46).

[3] The studies of Prentice Reeves and of Couvreux on the pupil, of Waller and, above all, of Haas on negative variation, have plainly demonstrated these facts.

of the distance between the value of the feeblest excitation perceptible and the strongest that acts without injury to the organism ; on the other, it is a function of the fineness of differential sensibility, which determines the number of steps and the rate of increase.

If this fineness of discrimination is observed under the most favourable conditions of medium excitation, it is greatest for light impressions, the differential fraction reaching 0·006. For raising weights it is about ten times less (0·06), and, for sound impressions, more nearly fifty times less (0·33).

However, if the variations of the intensity of the sensation are considered in relation to the variations in the intensity of the objective stimulus, it is necessary to take account of a very important factor, that of time. The laws of the times of sensations, therefore, have to be determined.

It is first learned that the sensation does not start instantly when the stimulus commences to act. The sensation is retarded, and the duration of this retardation, or the latency, is greater the weaker the stimulus.

Correlatively, the sensation does not cease as soon as the stimulus stops acting. It persists, and, in a symmetrical manner, the duration of the persistence increases as the intensity of the excitation decreases.[1]

Mathematical laws have been determined for luminous excitations, relating the duration of their latency and of their persistence to the intensity of the stimulus.[2]

By making the duration vary for the action of a stimulus

---

[1] A film which flickers when the light is very intense will cease to flicker, because of the increase of persistence, when the light is weaker. The variations of persistence are very great, in light impressions running from 5 to 120 thousandths of a second. After the cessation of the immediate persistence, consecutive negative and positive images are produced, corresponding to a series of oscillations gradually dying out (like those of a galvanometer when the current passing through it ceases abruptly).

[2] The approximate law of Ferry-Porter (the duration of the persistence is inversely proportional to the logarithm of the intensity) is not really satisfactory. The duration of the persistence is inversely proportional at low intensity, say at intensity of the first power (Charpentier indicates 0·5 power), the intensity varying with the experimental conditions (Law of Piéron).

of a given intensity, a correlative increase in the intensity of the sensation may be observed. Crossing the threshold after a certain retardation, the intensity apparently increases rapidly, goes beyond its level of stable equilibrium and then returns to this level, by an oscillation which resembles that of a galvanometer abruptly submitted to the action of an electric current. After reaching its equilibrium, it remains at this level for a certain time before slowly declining in consequence of a fatigue phenomenon.

When the stimulus ceases to act the sensation begins to decline, after a slight retardation, and disappears at the

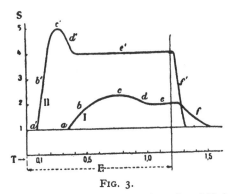

FIG. 3.

Diagram of the development of two sensations, I and II, in relation to time.

On the abscissa is shown the time (T) in seconds ; on the ordinate, the level of intensity of the sensations. The duration of the stimulus, (E), is indicated by the dotted line. For the more intense sensation, the time of latency (a) is shorter, the ascent (b) more rapid, the oscillation (c) more marked before the region of equilibrium (e), and the decline (f) more rapid.

end of a given time of persistence. See Fig. 3 for the diagram of the development of a sensation.

Time thus has an effect on the intensity of the excitation, at least during the quite brief first phase, which does not exceed a second except for stimuli near the threshold, and is clearly less than a hundredth of a second for intense stimuli. From this fact it is necessary to consider, for short excitations, not only the intensity of the stimulus (its amount of energy per unit of time), but also its quantity (the product of the intensity multiplied by the time, which is, for example, for light radiations of the same length of wave, a quantity of energy).

According to the law of Bloch, for short light excitations, this quantity of energy remains constant. It thus corresponds to a law found in photo-chemistry under the name of the law of Bunsen-Roscoe. It serves, however, only

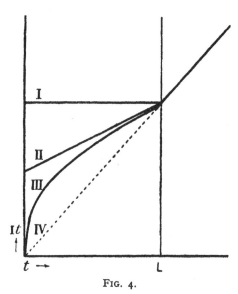

FIG. 4.

Diagram representing the different laws concerned with the relation between the quantity of threshold excitation (I*t*) and the duration of this excitation (*t*) for vision.

In I is shown the Law of Bloch, the quantity remaining constant; in II, the Law of Blondel and Rey (I$t=a+bt$; linear increase); in III, the Law of Piéron (I$t=at^n$; parabolic increase); in IV increase proportional to the time, which implies the invariability of the initial intensity. It is this which is verified beginning at L, representing the limit of summation for duration, called sometimes the " useful duration."

as an approximate law, like the law of Weber, valuable within the narrow limits of optimal excitations.

Blondel and Rey have shown that (as for the excitation of nerves, conforming to the law of Hoorweg-Weiss) the quantity of light stimulus necessary to reach the threshold increases regularly with the duration of the excitation and proportionally to the latter.

Representing on a diagram (see Fig. 4) the duration of excitations on the abscissa and the liminal quantity of light on the ordinate, in place of having a line parallel to the abscissa (Bloch's law) there would be a line which increases proportionally as the duration increases.

In reality this law is approximate and the process more complex. There is an ascent which is not in a straight line, but parabolic (Piéron's law). An increase in the quantity of energy for very short times has also been noticed, the graphic representation of which would then take the form of the S curve ; but this is a doubtful point.

The important fact is the loss which makes the summation of effects of the excitation more and more incomplete when this (using the same quantity of energy) is spread over a longer time. This is as if there were a leakage, or better stated, a resistance to overcome, which increased with time.

For short auditory excitations the same type of law has been established by P. Kucharski. But we still lack material for precise laws in relation to time for most of the sensations.

CHAPTER III

SPACE AND TIME

IN a perceptive experience, the analytic work of dissociation brings out certain common qualities in the numerous forms of sensory impressions. These may be systematized in a quite simple manner.

A dog runs and leaps around me ; I pass, while walking in the midst of the woods, at the side of a hill. The dog moves from right to left or from left to right, he jumps to various heights from the ground, he approaches or runs away, he runs in front of or behind me ; a tree is at my right, another at my left, they may be in front of or behind me, more or less distant ; some are higher, others lower, and, in the course of my walk, the distances and positions change.

Collective elaboration has reduced the complexity of these facts to four elementary perceptive qualities ; and the results were utilized above in verbally expressing these facts of perception. These four characteristics are four " directions " : before and after, left and right, forward and back, and high and low.

For each of these directions there is, on one hand, a sense of order, on the other, an extension. For the first one of these directions, the order is notably continuous and irreversible. If the dog had passed many times from my right to my left, the order before-after would include the positions right-left-right, etc., in a linear series registered once for all : that which had been before could not be an after-perception. If an analogous perception came after, we would know that it was not what had been there before, but another ; and the latter, being an after-perception, could not possibly be a before. We have no experience of any such reversal. In the series of the order right-left, we have on the contrary the experience of the inverse order, left-right.

In three directions, the sense of extension, the order is reversible. These are what are called the dimensions of space. The other direction is that of time. Movement can only be expressed as a function of space and time.

A. Perceptions of Time.

Like the other dissociated perceptive qualities, the temporal quality admits of quantitative appreciation, including an absolute threshold, a differential threshold, and comparisons of magnitude.   In all cases the estimates are interpreted differently according as they concern the amount of time in relation to a unified object of experience (the duration of which is estimated) or in relation to an interval between two individual experiences (that is to say, an interval of time), with an intermediate case of the interval between two slightly different aspects of a unified experience (the duration of the changing).

The absolute threshold will have to do with the minimum duration of a perceptive experience which is such that it ceases to appear instantaneous and has a temporal extent ; or with the minimum duration which must occur between two perceptive experiences for them to cease to appear simultaneous and manifest succession ; or, finally, with the minimum duration of a pause in order that it may be perceived in a changing process.

The limit of what is instantaneous is poorly understood and difficult to state precisely.   The threshold of pause has a practical value for the cinema, in which the successive images should continue for a time short enough for the change to appear continuous and not by jerks.   This is a variable threshold depending upon the conditions, the order of magnitude of which, however, is a few hundredths of a second.   Finally, the threshold of succession, or the limit of simultaneity, appears extremely variable.   It depends in part upon whether two or more impressions of a homogeneous sensory origin are observed.   If this is

G

done, the average threshold is from 5 to 10 hundredths of a second for vision, 1 to 2 hundredths for hearing or contact. Examples of average thresholds when the impressions belong to different senses are 5 to 7 hundredths of a second between vision and contact, 8 to 10 between vision and hearing, and 3 to 6 between hearing and contact. There is a large margin of uncertainty in the perception of the temporal order for heterogeneous impressions, with extreme variability and large errors, so that the apparent order of a series of events may be the reverse of the real order.[1]

When the temporal series of events is considered, it is necessary to take account, more than is generally done, more even than the relativists themselves have done, of processes of physiological transformation which are interposed between external events, or better, between the physical stimulus reaching the organism and the perceptive reaction. The differences due to the speed of sound or of light in the transmission of the signals until they reach the observer are taken account of, and yet it is apparently thought that at the time they reach the observer the perception follows instantaneously. But there are important times lost at the level of the sensory apparatus, retardations due to the nerve transmission and to connections at the relay centres. Depending upon the intensity and the nature of the excitation, the retardation may exceed a second or be reduced to two or three hundredths of a second. In fact, it is quite easy to set up,

---

[1] The difficulties in the appreciation of simultaneity appeared very soon to astronomers when they estimated the position of a star in the telescope in relation to the moment of the beat of a pendulum, called the eye and ear method. The estimate is very different, moreover, when one strives to follow a movement with the eye and when one submits to a visual stimulus. The positive experience of simultaneity, connected with a unified perceptive reaction, to a single act of observation, occurs only for homogeneous stimuli. With heterogeneous excitattions, there are always two distinct perceptive reactions. The simultaneity is inferred, with the possibility of reversing the order of two recognitions, depending upon one's inclination. A perception of simultaneity may be reached indirectly by proceeding to the motor reactions to two stimuli and giving attention to the kinæsthetic impressions. The two impressions of a homogeneous nature may then be made the object of a unified observation.

according to one's inclination, perceptive reactions for two events in an order of succession which is inverse to that of the peripheral stimuli.[1]

So far as concerns the perception of temporal magnitudes, it is necessary to consider separately those which involve intellectual appreciation, founded on a real calculation of time. Such durations exceed our direct perceptive capacity, our apprehension. There is quite a small limit to our capacity for direct, naïve perceptive reaction to durations. The limit appears to be 5 to 6 seconds at a maximum. Beyond this, arithmetical devices are utilized, though not always noticed.

Within the limits of direct perception, it is possible to determine the differential threshold for the estimation of the time which an excitation continues, or of the interval which elapses between two discontinuous excitations. It can be stated that there exists an optimal duration for which the comparisons are best. This is about a half-second. Moreover, at this optimum, the differential fraction remains sensibly constant, following Weber's Law. Its value is about a twentieth. Below this, short intervals are over-estimated, and above it, relatively long intervals are under-estimated.

In the perception of rhythms,[2] a little finer sensibility

---

[1] In the case of heterosensory stimuli, the influence of the attention can give an apparent precedence to a later stimulus, but then the reversal is easy. Again, when one stimulus in the same sensory field is notably weaker than another, it will appear clearly later when it is produced at the same time or even earlier. This is especially true in the visual field, because the physiological time lost preceding the perceptive reaction will be notably greater, the time diminishing in relation to the intensity of the stimulus.

[2] Rhythm implies repeated intervals of time, sensibly equal between the perceptions marking them off; and within these intervals the excitations may succeed each other very irregularly. It is an intensity accent especially which indicates the recurrence of the rhythm. This may be an objective accent or merely subjective, giving rise to a movement which " marks the rhythm." The intervals must be short enough to allow three repeated stimuli to succeed one another within the limits of the immediate perception of time. They never exceed 2 to 2·5 seconds.

Rhythm may be purely motor. In the spontaneous creation of rhythms, notable individual differences are recognized. A person has his own spontaneous rhythm : For example, an accentuation of the sixth stroke, the strokes succeeding each other with a frequency of 4 per second, would make an interval of 1·5 seconds for the group.

is noted for variations of the duration of periods, than if an isolated interval is considered, as in the preceding case.

B. *Spatial Perceptions*.

In all experience, no matter what its nature, the temporal qualities may be dissociated. It is not so evident that spatial qualities may be always dissociated. If " volume " is attributed to sounds—the spatial representations of which depend perhaps on association by analogy —and if, by acts of active orientation, the origin of an odour may be located in space, it is nevertheless true that spatial qualities belong especially to certain categories of sensation. These are vision and those relevant to mechanical excitations of the skin (contact and pricking sensations) and, in quite large measure, thermal excitations (warm and cold).

The retinal and cutaneous excitations are really endowed with a quality which changes with the place of the excitation in such a way that the differences perceived increase with the distance between the regions excited. This is true at least for excitations on one side of the body, with a certain similarity for symmetrical regions. This perception is often called, since Lotze, the " local sign," and may be dissociated from the total sensory experience. The qualitative excitations connected with the place of excitation imply, like all others, such as pitch or colour, a differential threshold which is expressed spatially.[1]   What

---

[1] There is a natural antagonism between the fineness of spatial discrimination and the capacity for "summation." For equal objective intensities, mechanical excitation on the skin or light on the retina produce a greater effect when the surface of application increases, *i.e.*, the absolute threshold is less for a more extended excitation. To produce summation, the effects of excitations on neighbouring points must be added in the same neurone. In the case of the fovea for each receptor cone there corresponds a neural ganglion. In the peripheral regions of the retina, numerous points of stimulation (200 on the average) enter into connection with a single cell station, hence there is a less discriminative capacity—the local sign requiring a single chain of neurones—and an increased capacity for summation. On an average the " Law of Ricco " may hold for the eye, according to which the summation is proportional to the square root of the surface stimulated.

is the mimimum distance between two excitations so that
the two are recognized as not being at the same point ?
In order to determine this threshold, it is well that the two
excitations should be successive. When they are simultaneous, three possibilities are present : 1. The impression
coming from both excitations aroused at the same time is
identical with that from a single excitation coming from
either one of the two when separately stimulated. 2. The
impressions are regarded as two excitations more or less
separate.   3. The excitations may be taken for a more
extended single excitation (the absolute spatial threshold,
the threshold of length, of extension, in a single direction).

The problem of the threshold of tactual acuity has been
studied with " Weber's compass," two points being applied
to the skin with a variable distance between them, and the
subject saying whether he perceived one or two points.
For a long time the question was badly formulated, so
that the answers depended upon the attitude of the
subjects, especially among children. In order to record
the impression of duality, it might be sufficient to have an
impression of unusual extension of the excitation, or it
might require the impression of an empty space (the
location of an intermediate non-stimulated local quality).
The difference between the thresholds founded on these
two criteria can be very great (2 mm. and 30 mm. according to Friedline).

The threshold of acuity is a function of the distribution
of the peripheral sensitive elements on the receiving
surface, the skin or retina,[1] and varies greatly with the
region stimulated. For the cutaneous surface, including
the mucous membranes, the threshold has values which
extend from 1 and 2 mm. at the point of the tongue and
at the ends of the fingers, to between 50 and 70 on the
back or thigh. On the retina the minimum threshold for

[1] Each fibre has its specific quality and can give location to a perception distinct from that which arouses the excitation of neighbouring
fibres. This is the anatomical and physiological limit of sensitivity.
If two excitations are carried exclusively on the same tactile fibre, the
local quality will be identical. This is true if the place and the extent
of the excitations are different. The same thing occurs for retinal cones
and the corresponding optical fibres, in relation to light or dark spots.

points is two microns (thousandths of a millimetre), subtending an angle of 30 seconds, and 0·33 (5 seconds) for lines lying end to end but not at an angle, or 7 according to Stratton. The so-called normal visual acuity is a little less. It corresponds to an angular value of a minute for the centre of the fovea ; at 25 degrees from the centre, the normal acuity is already reduced to a tenth, and, at 55 degrees, to a hundredth of its foveal value.

The thresholds of linear extension, retinal or cutaneous, refer to all directions which lie in a plane surface (or one which is sensibly plane), that is to say, which may be included in a space of two dimensions. For the third direction, other mechanisms are required.

Local quality is at the base of the still more complex processes of perception involved in a reaction called localization. This requires at least two spatial directions and generally three. A tactile excitation is recognized as occurring on a given region of the body, which will be designated verbally or by a gesture. The place of excitation will, for example, be touched.[1]

A retinal excitation in the right or left region, high or low, will cause the stimulating light or shadow to be referred to as left or right, low or high. The eye will turn so as to look in the direction of the stimulus, to project the image of the stimulating surface on the centre of the fovea. Furthermore, the surface originating the retinal excitation, will, within certain limits, be called near or far. In looking at it, the axes of the eyes will converge in such a manner as to form the image on the foveas of both eyes, and accommodation will occur so as to make the images clear.

Verbal reactions, intellectualized spatial perceptions, require training or education, as do most of the perceptive

---

[1] The error of active localization is less when the cutaneous region concerned serves more frequently for tactile explorations, and when it is richer in sensitive terminals. These generally go together. It is at a minimum on the fingers and the face. The error is smaller than for the threshold of discrimination, of acuity. The difference is more marked in the less sensitive regions. It is 20 mm. on the thigh or the back in place of 60 mm., while in the more sensitive tip of the tongue, it is 0·6 mm. instead of 1 mm.

reactions. But the mechanisms of congenital reactions, by reflex adaptation, provide for touching a point of the skin stimulated (scratching reflex), and for looking in the direction of a suddenly appearing bright surface, assuring suitable convergence and exact accommodation.

Local quality is, then, the point of departure for perceptive reflex reactions in the form of adapted movements.[1] It is these movements themselves which permit intellectualized spatial education. Movement gives spatial significance to the dissociable quality connected with the place of retinal or cutaneous excitation. It alone reveals the third dimension.

Space has interest and reality only as a place for motor activities, when it is necessary to reach an object placed high or low, at the right or at the left, far away and in front of another, near and behind, etc.

It is in connection with movement that tactile exploration provides for the appreciation of spatial extent,[2] under the aspect of distance or of homogeneous expansion (linear, on the surface, or especially in volumes). It consequently leads to the perception of form, which is a combination of extensions. A disturbance of ocular reflexes passes over into the visual notions of high and low, right and left, and also into those of near and far,[3] in spite of the difficulty of the " disparity " of the two retinas, which causes the impression of relief. This disparity is shown in the relative positions of the images of certain details of the visual picture on the two retinas, symmetrical points not being affected in an identical way ; or again by the discrepancy which would appear between images of the

---

[1] The reactions of monocular accommodation in relation to distance seem also to be connected to non-dissociated aspects of border-lines of light caused by the chromatic aberration of the optic system of the eye (Polack). In binocular vision, accommodation and convergence are closely associated.

[2] The estimates of the size of objects placed on the skin are very rough, but they gain precision by education, as among the blind. Static evaluations are based upon the memory of comparisons with dynamic evaluations.

[3] I have related some interesting observations by Gordon Holmes on this aspect of the matter in my *Thought and the Brain* (in the International Library).

two retinas, if they were superimposed with the centres of
the foveas and the horizontal axes coinciding.

Normally, certain objects are perceived as forward and
others as back, since the point of an image fixated by the
eyes is or is not perceived at this real distance, depending
upon its relation to the point of regard (the image of which
is found on the corresponding symmetrical positions in
the two retinas). This visual perception of distance is
thus a function of the side and of the amount of disparity
between the images of objects on the corresponding
regions of the two retinas. There is a threshold of disparity, of discrepancy, directly perceptible, and a much
finer threshold perceptible under the aspect of the reaction
of relief,[1] or an absolute threshold of extension, of spatial
magnitude traceable to the third dimension.

A more marked contrast between the thresholds for
direct and indirect perception is found in auditory localization. If sounds do not have evident spatial extension,
an auditory knowledge of the place of their origin is always
acquired, including directions to the right or left, high or
low, and the approximate distance. While remaining
immovable, one has a clear perception of the lateral origin
of a sound. This is quite rough when it is based upon the
difference in intensity at the level of the two ears, and
very precise when it is based upon a difference in time
between the starting of the excitation in the two sets of
auditory apparatus (the two mechanisms having been
experimentally dissociated). Half of a ten-thousandth
of a second is sufficient to reach the threshold of lateral-
ization of a sound. This threshold is that of the reflex of
ocular exploration of the side where the source of the
sound is found. The knowledge of this reflex is translated
into the form of a spatial perception. On the other hand,
as we have indicated previously, the direct perception of
an auditory succession requires a difference of about a
hundredth of a second, more than a hundred times longer.

---

[1] An effect of stereoscopic relief may be obtained with a disparity
amounting to an angular distance of only 3 seconds, corresponding to a
linear distance of 0·2 of a micron ; in order to perceive a distance between
two points requires at a minimum 30 seconds, or ten times more.

An entire series of other spatial perceptions is exclusively dependent upon taking cognizance of reflex motor reactions, especially ocular reactions. The isolated excitations of the apparatus of the labyrinths do not directly produce dissociable perceptions, but they arouse adaptive reactions of equilibrium and compensating ocular movements, which are themselves perceived under the form of a displacement of the body in space or of the displacement of objects in relation to the body. These labyrinthine excitations occur in the ampulla of the semi-circular canals in case of rotations of the body and in the utriculus and sacculus in translations of the body. The labyrinth sense, which has only spatial value, gives rise only to reflex perceptive reactions. The analysable spatial perception, which may be intellectualized, is closely related to the execution of reactional movements, and to the impressions which result from them.

C. *Spatio-Temporal Perceptions : Movement.*

In movement the spatial and temporal elements are combined in a unified experience, which has speed as its proper characteristic. This is the relation of a spatial magnitude to a temporal magnitude. Both absolute and differential thresholds for speed may be determined for various movements, including movement of the whole body, partial movement of a segment of the body, movement of an object kept in view (this amounts to a movement of the eye), and the relative movement of an object in relation to the body when the body remains quiet. This last corresponds to the rapidity of change of local quality with an interpretation of this change as spatial extension.

So far as movements of the body in space are concerned,[1] they are not directly perceived when they are uniform. This is a particular case of the general relativity of movement. Only positive or negative accelerations can be

[1] Visual, tactual and other sensory combinations often permit an inference of displacement.

noticed, and then only through the reactions which they excite.[1]

Nevertheless a uniform rotation about an axis, producing a centrifugal force, may be perceived, the perception taking a static form, especially as an apparent inclination of the vertical in the direction of the resultant of the centrifugal force and gravity.

The absolute and differential thresholds of the perception of movement of a member of the body have been very little studied under the specific aspect of speed. The absolute threshold implies a minimum quantity of movement, that is to say, of the space traversed or of the duration of the movement ; one of the elements implies the other when the speed is determined. The spatial and temporal components of movement have been studied separately, in conformity with the traditional plan of our results. In particular the smallest angular displacement which is perceptible has been determined for each articulation of the body (Goldscheider). This runs from a fifth of a degree to about a degree and a half.

As to movements of the eyes, it is known that a very slow movement of 1' in a second is perceived, but this case includes visual impressions on the retina. In the dark, eye movements are much more difficult to perceive, even with a speed thirty times greater.

[1] An acceleration of a few centimetres per second is perceived in movements of translation.

THE PERCEPTIVE REACTION AND ITS STAGES

THE adaptation of conduct to various objects and various situations is regulated by sensory experiences which are generally very incomplete and fragmentary. I hear my name called in a certain complex quality of voice, and at once have the reaction that I am meeting a friend, the reaction which comes for a definite friend more or less warmly received. In the perception, there is an anticipation of experience which corresponds to a mechanism of conditioned reflexes. When the mouth waters at the sight of an agreeable fruit, there is, by anticipation, the normal reaction from tasting the savoury morsel. The perception will be released by a fragment of a sensory experience which has been less or more common, depending upon which preparatory attitude is better suited to the nature of the object perceived. If I am waiting for a friend in a reception room, the noise of an opening door will suffice to excite at once the perceptive conduct.

As a result of this anticipation, the perception will be subject to more or less error, to illusion. For example, when I read in a text one word in place of another less common or more unexpected, the perception is released by the appearance of certain typical letters common to two words which are of the same length.

Special experimental studies of reading by Javal, by Erdmann and Dodge, by Huey, and others have furnished highly interesting results bearing on the process of perception.

Whenever we read, our eye, without our knowing it at all, fixates at a certain number of places for short pauses, in the course of which vision occurs, and moves by jumps between these successive pauses, the jumps being so quick

that they are ignored and do not produce any visual
perception.

When reading an easy text in my native language with
lines about 10 centimetres long (64 letters) in 7-point type,
I have counted six pauses, in 9-point type (47 letters), four
or sometimes five pauses. The duration of each pause
was from two to three-tenths of a second. The speed of
rapid reading for a skilled person is about 50 letters a
second.[1]

In reading, it is very certain that the perception of words
is a unified reaction which does not include the discrimination of individual letters. This reaction may be speeded
up by practice. It is released by more and more vague
and incomplete sensory impressions, as may be noted from

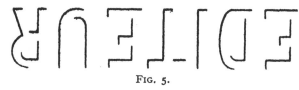

FIG. 5.

Look at the figure and then turn the page upside down and look again.

the adjoining figure, in which some rather chaotic lines,
when they are presented conveniently, are immediately perceived as constituting a French word (Fig. 5). A reader may
proceed more slowly because his eye stops more often and
longer at a time along the line. This gives more definite
sensations, and the field of vision is only slightly extended.
The eye takes in at a time only 3 or 4 letters instead of
10 or 12, as though for the careful correction of proof
which requires noting every incorrect letter. If understanding the phrases becomes difficult, as with a foreign
language, less common words or less common associations
of words, the number of eye-stops increases per line, the
number of letters perceived at each stop diminishes, and
the reading is notably slower because of the multiplication

[1] A trained blind person reading Braille characters with his fingers
reaches 13 letters a second.

and lengthening of the pauses. The length of the pauses may reach and even exceed half a second each.

The usual perception is quick, like every reaction to a frequently repeated excitation. The crude sensory impression is scarcely passed when the perceptive reaction develops through attitudes, sentiments, movements, verbal expressions or otherwise.

This shows clearly in " tachistoscopic " experiments having to do especially with reading. These permit groups of consonants, of separate words, or of short phrases to appear for a very short time. It is found that a length of exposure which will permit 6 consonants to be recognized, is sufficient for the perception of a dozen letters grouped in syllables, nearly 15 letters in words, and about twice that number if grouped in a short phrase. This is due to the greater familiarity of the perception.

There is anticipation of a familiar response, but for this reason the wrong response may be favoured. An impression to which we are not accustomed, having a certain similarity to a common impression, will start up the familiar perceptive reaction just as the latter itself would. One word will thus be substituted for another, as we have mentioned. The mistake will be corrected or not, according as the erroneous perceptive reaction leads or does not lead to attitudes or acts which are obviously in disagreement with later events. A word taken for another will arouse either another meaning which persists because more or less compatible with the following text, or it will, on the contrary, cause the reader to turn back and correct it because of the contradictions and absurdities which arise from the original error.

I think that I see a friend in the crowd, and I remain convinced that I have seen him if he disappears at once ; but I would have recognized my error if I had started to shake hands with him, because the astonishment of the person accosted would have made me realize that I had been deceived by a certain resemblance.

In cases where a mistake may later be practically checked (an account of an accident, for example) under frequently repeated conditions, the mistake is by degrees completely corrected. It will persist if it cannot be checked at all.

Errors of perception often carry with them corresponding anticipations. This explains the practical need of sufficiently quick reactions, in order, for example, on the approach of an automobile when one crosses the street, that the adaptation to the size, the distance, the speed, etc., may take place by continuing at a normal pace, running, or stopping. This evaluation takes place by behaviour that may be described as determined. When a marble is placed between the ends of the index and middle fingers crossed (illusion of Aristotle), we have the perceptive reaction of two marbles because never, under ordinary conditions, have we had experience of a single object giving similar contacts on the sides of the two fingers here concerned. Inversely, contacts on the sides of the fingers normally adjacent arouse the perception of a single object (illusion of Rivers). But new education, by repeated experiences with the fingers crossed, will build up a better adapted perception.

Some more elementary sensory experiences also cause illusions which are then more tenacious. For example, the points of a compass kept a constant distance apart and drawn over the skin seem to approach each other or to separate. This depends upon whether the sensitivity of the skin for spatial discrimination is more or is less fine. The estimation of the separation of the points is conditioned in great part by the liminal unit of spatial extension for each region.

Many classical visual illusions are connected with retinal diffusions, motor reflexes of the eyes, etc. They imply the intervention of relatively elementary processes. We may instance the illusion of Zoellner, in which there is an apparent separation of two parallel lines crossed by oblique lines in an inverse direction to the illusion ; the Müller-Lyer illusion of an apparent lengthening or shortening of lines ending in angles extended outwards or inwards, etc. One direction of experimental study of very many forms of illusion has been much emphasized in the endeavour to make their conditions and their mechanisms precise; namely, a general tendency to accentuate the characteristics of objects and of individualized images, almost to the point of caricature. The explanation of illusions is thus sought in the attempt to trace them to a unifying assimilation to objects; or, on the other hand, to a separating opposition (contrast).

But it must not be forgotten that illusion, like every perceptive reaction, is conditioned by a veritable complex, involving attitudes, necessary preliminary experiences, and a diversity of sensory impressions.

Let us consider the illusion of movement which arises whenever two points appear one after the other in the field of vision and a short distance apart. A point is seen to move from the first place towards the second. Various elementary conditions of sensory experience come in : the distance between the points, the interval between their appearance, the light, etc. ; but also quite other conditions. If a model is seen following a similar course, if the points consist of two pictures of a football, with a picture, at the side, of a foot which kicks it, the movement is then perceived under elementary conditions when it would not be seen except for these influences.

This shows that the perception is a total reaction to an entire situation, which can become the object of a later analysis, but which does not consist of an intellectual synthesis, impregnated with logic, as all the classical theories of perception have believed.[1]

The original datum of perception, in the biological domain, is the objective reality to which it must, in order to survive, adapt itself. The elementary characteristics of this datum acquire perceptive value only so far as an artistic, literary, scientific or philosophical task, that is

[1] The perceptive reaction, when it is developed under the associative form, may imply an analysis followed by a new synthesis, but it then results from special training. Whenever a person is submitted repeatedly to introspective tasks, the perception changes, expands, slows up, becomes an act of discursive thought, the more capable of justifying the classical theories in that it really results from training which is governed by these same theories.

to say, a task of social origin, requires their analytic dissociation. In regard to "illusion," what should be explained is, in general, not the illusion itself, but its eventual correction. It is not normal to perceive forms, extensions, colours, and brightnesses with exactness, but only to recognize objects in such a manner as to react correctly when face to face with them, and quickly enough for the reaction not to come too late.

The general law of what we shall call *perceptive individualization* is that all sensory experience gives place normally to perception in the measure in which it permits an object or a situation to be individualized so as to adapt a definite form of attitude and conduct to it. Among civilized men this behaviour may be limited to an associative activity of a form more or less exclusively verbal, to a purely mental attitude.

This individualization appears to be founded on earlier experiences and to arise through the empirical gropings which are known in animal psychology as the method of trial and error.[1] We shall now consider some examples of individualization in the field of visual perception.

1. *The colour of objects, brightness and the " albedo."*— A grey paper placed in full light is much more bright, more " white," than white paper placed in a shadow ; nevertheless the first is called grey and the second white. This depends on the fact that the perceptive character, white or grey, is only a means of individualizing an object, of recognizing it under varying brightnesses. The appreciation of the reflecting property of an object is known scientifically as the " albedo." This, and not the real brightness, which is essentially variable, is of interest in determining

[1] The notion of *Form* (*Gestalt*) developed by an interesting and active school of German philosophy (Koehler, Koffka, Wertheimer) corresponds in this particular, that the perception is a response to a situation individ- alized as a whole. Very many experiments, inspired by the theory, have clearly established the part played by general conditions—of the Gestalt—on various quite definite perceptions of extension, movement, brightness, etc. But the theory goes beyond the facts. It gives to Form as such a value which is questionable, and it seeks to discover the causes, not in the acquisition of experience—individual or ancestral— but in the physiological organization and also in the laws of physical chemistry (Koehler).

the individual object, in recognizing the object as integrated in our activity. On the other hand, the general lighting is the object of an individualized perception (depending on whether the room is light or dark) ; which perception will be based on seeing grey papers and white papers, and, in fact, all objects in general.[1] It is difficult to learn to appreciate the absolute brightness of a surface which is a function of its own reflecting power and of general illumination brightness ; but this, in its turn, may become a perceptive task. We will then individualize this absolute brightness as in photometry, for example.

Before training vision for brightness, these fundamental facts are utilized either in an individualizing perception of objects (in which the constancy extends to all properties, including the albedo), or in a perception of variations of clearness, which permits us to appreciate, for example, that the dusk is coming.

In the same way, we speak of objects as red, green or blue, in so far as we individualize them according to their colour. Under conditions of light in which their colours really vary, and in which a scrupulous painter will distinguish the play of various blends, the objects will remain red, green or blue. Moreover, the public, lacking the artistic education which trains to individualize colour, often considers as fantastic in a picture the colourings of trees, of the sky and of the most common objects. When face to face with the painting, the public's critical, analytic attitude is very different from that which it takes when facing the actual subject represented.

2. *Extension and Form.*—The perceptions of size behave in the same manner as those of brightness and colour. The size of objects is a characteristic which permits their individualization. Just as white or grey or black is judged to be such under different illuminations, because of

[1] Among animals which react in a different way to general illumination and to the albedo of their background, the same dissociation may be noticed. On a dark surface under an intense light, some crustaceans take on a dark colour ; under a feeble light, they assume a clear, transparent condition just like that when on a white surface under a strong light.

H

a simultaneous perceptive reaction to the real brightness of the surface and to the intensity of the illumination, so the size of an object is a reaction to the dimension of the retinal image, *i.e.*, to its angular size, and to its distance, known or assumed. With the same image we may have the impression of a small or of a large object, as, when behind a car window, we believe that we have seen a fly near at hand or a cow in the distance.

When objects are at a short distance, and one which may be perceived by the degree of convergence of the eyes, we appreciate the size of the object as of the dimension which corresponds to the angular size of the retinal image projected to the distance of the plane on which the eyes are fixed through their convergence (Law of Giraud-Teulon). This estimation is such that, if the ocular convergence is artificially increased or diminished, this is enough to change the apparent size of the objects and to produce experimentally a micropia or macropia.[1] In a similar way, people in a drawing take on the size which corresponds to their apparent distance (see Fig. 6). In the case of drawings, however, we do not adopt quite the same attitude as in the presence of the real scenes.

The appreciation of size by itself, its individualization, requires training, as does also the correct perception of form, which is necessary for making designs.

With a child, and with an adult who has not studied design, all wheels are round, although not one in a thousand

[1] The phenomena of "shadows in relief," the cinema attraction which has amused many people, affords a curious example of the truth of this law. Viewed through green and red glasses, a single shadow-object on the screen is produced by the fusion of the green shadow seen by one eye and the red shadow seen by the other. This shadow-object is seen to approach and to diminish in size at the same time when the object throwing the shadows is brought near to the sources of the red and green lights. The lights are separated more than the eyes, so that the shadows on the screen diverge, and the more they diverge the larger they grow. The curious incongruity of the appearance is due to the fact that, in order to maintain the fusion of the shadows, the eyes are forced to converge more. The plane on which the eyes are fixated then approaches them, and the shadow in relief seems to be a real object localized at the distance of this plane. The shadow-object thus appears to approach, but is also perceived as smaller on this nearer plane of convergence, according to the Law of Giraud-Teulon, which explains the absurd result of the appearance.

is seen round, and although for the eyes they are a variety of ellipses. Thus not forms but wheels are individualized.[1]

3. *Distance and Relief.*—A whole series of characteristics of impressions is translated into perceptions of distances, arousing appropriate activities, the importance of which is evident. In order to avoid an obstacle, to dip a pen in the ink, to go upstairs, to pick up a glass, reactions to the individualized distances of objects are required.

Among the many factors which contribute to the correct reactions among normal individuals possessing binocular vision, is " retinal disparity." This is the discrepancy

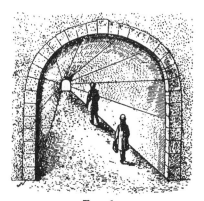

FIG. 6.

Note that the person in front is, in reality, shorter.

between the images of objects in the two eyes as they would appear on a combined retina formed by the superposition of the receptive surfaces of the two eyes. When fixing, at a definite distance, a point, the images of which are formed at the centres of the two retinas, nearer objects throw their images to the outside of the centre, more distant objects to the inside, the divergence increasing with their distance from the point fixated. This produces

[1] J. Payot has well emphasized these characteristics of perception : " Stop before the window of a jeweller : all the watches are presented in very different perspective, but you see them as if you looked at them all perpendicularly. . . . You see a tree in its green colour even when it is badly lighted by a gas light in the street." (*Revue philosophique*, June, 1891, pp. 630–631.)

the perceptive reaction of relief. It is artificially reproduced in the stereoscope, which makes us see two different images, one for each eye, presenting the proper disparities.

Innumerable researches, stimulated by philosophical problems often very badly stated, have been devoted to the perception of relief. Here again, it must not be forgotten that the perceptive reaction, set up by certain sensory impressions, is always a reaction to a total situation and that repeated experiences are able to modify it.

Whenever a " pseudoscopic " effect is produced, as by presenting in a stereoscope the left-eye image to the right eye and the right-eye image to the left eye, the apparent distances and the relief are reversed. This is clearly seen, for example, with geometrical figures of cones.[1] But, if the experiment is tried with photographs of the country and of complex scenes, it is realized that the reversal of relief does not always take place, in spite of the inversion of the retinal disparities. When a very tall person is beside a small tower, according to the natural images, it is difficult to obtain the reverse effect with the stereoscopic pictures. It is not possible generally to see the tower in front and the person behind, permitting the perceptive reaction to agree with the retinal disparity, or at least this effect can only be brought about by long and special training. It is never possible to succeed in reversing the human face.

4. *Movement and Speed.*—An object moves while we follow its movement with the eye ; we perceive its movement has occurred at a certain speed. If our eye remains still, the displacement of the image on the retina also produces a perception of movement and an appreciation of its speed. But, for the same movement, the speed perceived is very different in the two cases. If our eye remains quiet the movement appears very rapid ; if our eye follows it, there is an apparent slowing up which is

---

[1] There are so-called reversible figures, which, when they are stared at for a long time, appear sometimes to be concave and at others to project.

very noticeable.[1] This is probably due to the fact that, under the usual conditions, we fail to follow a movement with the eye only when the movement becomes very rapid. It follows that, if the eye is artificially held still, our education not being complete, over-estimation is produced. The effect on our appreciation is like that of a speed too rapid to be followed by a movement of the eye.

Suddenly appearing movements may indeed be perceived when impressions succeed each other on different points, as happens whenever an object—a thrown ball, for example —moves between two positions too quickly to be followed by the eye or to give time to perceive the intermediate images on the retina. The whole excitation, however, must have a minimum duration, relative to its intensity, in order to produce a sensation.

For continuous movements, it is, nevertheless, the speed of ocular movements of pursuit which assures their exact appreciation.

Here again, the perceptive reaction excited by the movement of the eye is in reality conditioned by an entire complex, since the same movement, depending upon the circumstances, will be perceived differently. It may be perceived as a movement of the eye, as in reading, for example, in which case the images change regularly when the eye moves; as a movement of an object, the same point of an object being fixated while the eye moves; or again, depending upon whether the eyes are closed or open, either as a movement of the body (during the dizziness which follows a suddenly arrested rotation, in which the nystagmus, when the eyes are closed, makes us believe that we are turning in a reverse direction), or as a movement of objects (when we hold the eyes open after the rotation and the change of images, due to the involuntary

[1] If a band of numbers or letters is attached to a rotating drum, the speed of rotation is appreciated by trying to read distinctly the letters or numbers. This implies that the movement is accompanied by the eyes in order to permit a stable image, necessary for reading, to be formed on the retina. Whenever the vision becomes indistinct, for example through the diminution of the light, the eye no longer functions, and the movement appears to be very much accelerated, at least three or four times as fast.

nystagmus, which is identical with that which would be produced in the course of a voluntary displacement of the eyes, makes us think that the world is turning round and passing before our unmoved eyes).

Ocular movement thus, according to circumstances, gives rise to very different types of individualized perceptions of movement.

We would find, in other sensory fields, plenty of examples analogous to these. We may cite the appreciation of " weight." Except among merchants who individualize this characteristic,[1] weight is really a recognition of densities which serve as the specific elements for the individualization of objects. It is very certain that a pound of lead is heavier than a pound of feathers, because it is the lead and the feathers which we individualize in speaking of " heavier," and not the pound. In the same way, grey paper in the sunlight remains more grey than white paper in a shadow.

Like the movements of the eyes, movements of the arms are perceived under different aspects depending upon the complex of the moment. Although a separate movement of one arm appears as a simple lateral displacement, this displacement to the side is not perceived when there is a simultaneous movement of both arms : when these converge or diverge, only the separation or approach is perceived ; when the movement is made in the same direction with both arms and the eyes are closed, it is the body

[1] The individualization of the sensation, which is necessary for a subject submitting to experiments intended to measure the differential sensibility in order to verify, for example, Weber's Law, is not always attained. There is produced what Titchener calls " stimulus error." This error is a return to the natural attitude. If a subject is asked to determine a weight half way between two others, he may seek a sensation of middle intensity, or—what is natural, but constitutes an error according to Titchener—a weight which the balance will show is half way between. If there is not an objective standard, what is only an impression is confused with what is a characteristic of the object. This happens when a scale of greys is established, for example, since the physical appreciation of brightnesses has remained subjective, as has also the notion of light.

which appears to be inclined and in the opposite direction (Michotte).

The same complexes as occur in binocular vision between size, form, and direction or distance, are encountered again in binaural hearing between the intensity and the apparent volume of sounds and their localization.

Perceptive reactions are excited by masses of sensory impressions. Certain of these elements are individualized and become real objects of perception. Others entirely escape from all effort of analytic discrimination, as does the extraordinarily short interval of time separating the moments when each ear has been affected by a sound, an interval which can be known only in the form of a lateral direction of the source of the sound.

But, in all cases, whether analysis is or is not possible, what may be called the " syncretic " reaction of perception is primitive and natural. This is well shown by the study of higher animals and children. A detached " sensation " arises only from analytic education. Just the reverse has been believed, namely, a synthetic perceptive construction founded on simple sensory elements. This most serious error of psychology has caused it to follow absolutely artificial problems like that of how things are seen right side up,[1] the priority of corresponding points in retinal rivalry, the notion of externalization or of objectivity, etc.

[1] The retinal image is only an element in the perceptive complex, which expresses itself in attitudes and motor reactions. The axes of spatial reference are biologically defined by the directions of gravity and of the gaze ; the notions of right and left have become very complicated from social usage because regulated by variable conventions.

CHAPTER V

CONGENITAL EQUIPMENT AND MNEMONIC ACQUISITION

THE FIXATION OF MEMORIES

MOST perceptive reactions of a spatial nature are congenitally predetermined, as we have noted. The localization of a cutaneous excitation, of a light or sound stimulation, is defined by motor reflexes of the limbs, of the head, and of the eyes, disclosed among the new-born in a very precocious fashion. But, if the reflexes continue to be produced under the same circumstances there will never be that adaptive plasticity characteristic of psychological functions, which requires the acquisition of experience. Whether congenital perceptive reactions were first acquired by trial and error or by chance variations in the physical-chemical structure of the germs, is a problem like all questions of origin which escapes investigation.[1] But we observe, during the life of an individual, the pre-existing reactions developing, becoming more perfect and more flexible, and the birth of innumerable new reactions.

The total reaction to an excitant, whether adapted or not, is an experience, the influence of which tends to conserve, and to contribute to the amelioration and progress of conduct. A perception, which usually represents mnemonic acquisitions put to work, is always retained as a memory.

The processes of memory appear in elementary planes

---

[1] Biologists in general refuse to-day to admit the inheritance of acquired characteristics, of adaptive modifications arising in the course of an individual's life. But there are some results which point to the hereditary transmission of certain individual modes of behaviour.

of life, where the mnemonic persistence of rhythms repeated for a long time may be observed among plants, lower animals, and even in single organs among the most highly evolved beings. There is also habitually the associative transfer of stimulating power from one excitation to another which accompanies it, and especially to one which precedes it. The fundamental law of biological anticipation thus emerges. According to this, the sign preceding a harmful effect which aroused a reaction of defence is sufficient to again set up this reaction, thus favouring the protection of the organism.[1]

In the conditioned reflexes studied by Pavlov are found the definite laws of nerve action in associative transfer, which is the fundamental type of mnemonic acquisition. For example, the more the association is repeated between the direct excitant which arouses a congenitally adapted reaction, and any other stimulus which becomes by transfer a conditioned excitant arousing the same reaction, the more prompt, efficient, stable, and lasting, will be the power acquired by the latter to start the reflex.

On the other hand, the longer the time which elapses after the last association, the weaker becomes the power to arouse a reflex. There is a gradual automatic disappearance of acquired connections. At a certain time the power peculiar to a conditioned excitant seems to have disappeared, and the associated stimulus becomes wholly ineffective ; but there is still in reality a latent power, since a new association gives the excitant a higher effectiveness than it would have from a new stimulus.

Along with the automatic disappearance of the acquired connection between the two stimuli, there may be a more rapid artificial weakening, resulting from the play of an active inhibitional factor. If the action of the conditioned excitant is stimulated many times in succession without the association of the other excitant from which it draws its force for generating reflexes, this force decreases

---

[1] The animals which live attached to rocks in the tidal zone, show defence reactions against drying, which occur before the falling tide has uncovered them. Baldwin has noted facts of anticipation acquired in the first stages of an infant's development.

very rapidly, more rapidly the more frequent the repetition, although, if it had not been made to act many times, this conditioned excitant would still have had all its force. The effacing action itself has all the characteristics of a mnemonic acquisition, that is to say, of an actually inhibitive experience. The proof is that, if a certain time is allowed to elapse after the successive actions of the isolated conditioned excitant, which, from the fact of spontaneous effacement, would have decreased in power, nevertheless its reflexogenic power recovers a greater effectiveness. Again, the more recent inhibiting action is partially effaced, and more rapidly than the action of the reflexogenic transfer which is already old ; the inhibiting action which had become greater than the latter is found to be less after a certain time, since both have decreased, but with unequal rapidity.

It was by counting the drops of saliva secreted in the course of the conditioned reflex that Pavlov and his students were able to appreciate the force of the reflexogenic power of the stimulus.

Moreover, numerous reactions of animals studied by methods of " training " have also revealed these fundamental laws of associative transfer and acquired inhibition. They have been established for higher animals by American psychologists, including Thorndike.

Facts of the same order have also been observed among lower animals. Molluscs and worms retreat into their shells or into their tubes when a shadow is thrown on them. If, after the shadow, a shock or a prick occurs, the reaction regularly takes place ; but if nothing happens, the reaction to the shadow quickly ceases to be produced. This is an acquired inhibition, conditioned in Pavlov's sense.[1]

Inhibition weakens with time, and the reaction re-

---

[1] The phenomenon called " habituation," of becoming accustomed to a situation, studied in man, appears to respond, in the sphere of the reflexes, to analogous mnemonic mechanisms. The progressive diminution of nystagmus excited by repeated rotations has been studied, and the loss of the habituation occurring with time, when the experiences have ceased (Dodge).

appears. When the inhibition has apparently completely disappeared it is acquired anew more quickly, however, than the first time. This reveals the existence of a latent effect from the first acquisition.

By obtaining a certain inhibition effect in relation to the time elapsed since the last experience, it is possible to investigate what economies may be made in the number of repetitions, of necessary responses. The amount of this mnemonic trace is evaluated numerically, its regular decrease with time is followed, and a law of spontaneous loss, of forgetting, is obtained. But this law—with constants for different times—is found to be the same when the loss of verbal memory is studied in man[1] by an analogous method (the method of economy used by Ebbinghaus).

All the results relative to the associative transfer of a reflexogenic power are found again when one examines the mnemonic acquisitions of verbal associations, but these are naturally also more rich. By experimental studies the conditions of simple and well-defined fixation are examined. The experimenter reads to a subject, or causes him to read, a series of non-sense syllables—or of numbers, of letters, of words, etc., and the subject has to remember and repeat them.

The progress of the fixation is followed in relation to the readings, the influence exercised on the progress is examined for the intervals between the readings, for the effect of efforts to recite, for the number of elements to be retained, for the nature of the latter, for the disturbing action of other directed efforts, etc.

Evidence has been provided of a very considerable effect favourable to fixation, which comes from effort, interest and certain emotions (although others, intense emotion in particular, inhibit fixation) ; the effect of the nature of the elements to be remembered (words being more easily retained than non-sense syllables) ; the effect, varying

---

[1] This law corresponds to a hyperbolic decrease of the amount of the mnemonic impression. It may be stated in this form : The trace varies inversely to a fractional power of the elapsed time (Piéron).

with individuals, of the mode of presentation (certain people memorizing more quickly what they hear, others what they read with their eyes), or of the time of day when the memorizing is attempted.

As to the number of elements to be acquired the following observations have been made. When this number is small it is possible to obtain a correct repetition without true mnemonic acquisition, thanks to a simple persistence of the perception, to a capacity for apprehension. Thus individuals will repeat 5 or 7 or 10 numbers, after a single hearing, but forget them at once ; a few moments suffice for losing them completely. If we add one or two numbers more, they cannot be repeated except after a true memorizing, after repeated readings. But this time the acquisition will last, there will be a true memory.

Between the capacity for immediate repetition and fixation there is a definite hiatus. Increasing the number of elements to be retained makes the fixation more difficult and the difficulty progressively increases, corresponding to the square of the number of elements to be retained (Foucault, D. O. Lyon). It requires four times as long to retain forty numbers as twenty. Diamandi learned 15 numbers in 75 seconds, and 30 in 260 seconds, nearly four times the time ; but he learned 100 numbers in 25 minutes and 200 numbers in 135 minutes, more than five times the time. The law of the square is then only an approximate law, for retention of medium difficulty.

But, if after each reading, the proportion of correct repetitions is noted, it is found in all cases that the progress of the acquisition, with some irregularity, follows a quite similar curve. The progress begins by accelerating, then it slows down. For example, for a series of 25 numbers, 5 are retained after the first reading, 13 (+8) after the second, 19 (+6) after the third, 22 (+3) after the fourth, 24 (+2) after the fifth and 25 (+1) finally after the sixth. The progress of fixation, like all phenomena of organic growth which we know, tends to follow an S-shaped curve.

The rapidity of progress, however, in relation to the number of readings, depends much upon the distribution of the readings. If they occur one after the other without any intervals between, the total time for the learning may be less than if intervals are introduced, but the effort necessary for retention is greater, and the number of readings required is very much higher.

For example, in order to learn 20 numbers, a person requires 11 readings one after the other, 6 when an interval of five minutes separates the readings, and 5 when the interval is longer, but more than 5 if the interval is more than a day.

This fact shows—in addition to the possible intervention of certain phenomena of fatigue—that the mnemonic acquisition is not instantaneous, but there is a latent development, a period when it matures. This is what

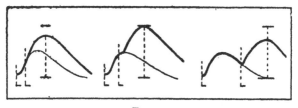

FIG. 7.

Graph showing that the total effect of two mnemonic acquisitions should be at a maximum for a certain interval between the two acquisitions, which corresponds to the duration of the complete maturation of the first acquisition, when the second comes at the moment that a phase of decline is about to follow this maturation.

was observed to show itself in another connection, with shorter times, in the fixation of an inhibiting process among molluscs reacting to a shadow, to which we have referred. When an optimal interval is adopted, when each effort of fixation comes at the moment when the preceding has attained all its effect, but before effacement has begun its work, the result sought is obtained most economically (see Fig. 7).

After this maturation the mnemonic acquisition really tends to keep its force for some time and then to decrease automatically. Then again, when numbers learned can no longer be repeated, they may still be relearned more quickly than the first time. This economy affords a measure of the strength of the trace left by the first acquisition.

This is a case where we again learn from our experiments. In the acquisition of equal series of numbers it is found that there is a saving of 85 per cent. in relearning one series after an interval of 2 weeks, of 64 per cent. after 4 weeks for another series ; 40 per cent. after 2 months for a third series ; and 25 per cent. after 4 months for a fourth series.

Automatic forgetting, when it commences, after a few days, develops at first quite rapidly, then its pace slows up

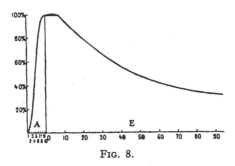

FIG. 8.

Graph showing the development, in relation to time, of a mnemonic acquisition, according to experimental values from memorizing a series of 50 numbers.

The phase of acquisition, represented by A, involved ten repetitions at the rate of one a day. The phase of disappearance is shown by E. On the abscissa is shown the number of days elapsing after the fixation. After 90 days the persistence still represents 40% of the initial value.

more and more. It develops as a function of a fractional power of the time, as we have indicated above.

The history of a memory, shown on a very condensed time scale, might be inscribed on a graph which could be superimposed on that of organic reactions, such as a simple muscular contraction produced by a series of successive nerve impulses (see Fig. 8).

But besides the spontaneous loss there exist certain positive influences of effacement, artificial inhibitions of mnemonic acquisitions.

For example, after having learned a series of numbers or syllables, if another is learned, the second effaces in part the memory of the first[1] ; moreover, the effect is greater the closer is the similarity between the two acquisitions. A series of numbers effaces the memory of another series of numbers more than it will a series of syllables or words.

The effacing action of a new acquisition will be weaker, however, the longer the time which elapses ; that is to say, the old memory will become more stable than directly after the effacing acquisition. Indeed, the latter will automatically die out more quickly than the old acquisition and its own action will be proportionately less, since the curve of spontaneous forgetting shows a rapid loss of memory when the decline commences, and a slower and slower loss with time ; the acquisition causing the efface-ment is in the period of rapid decline, the old acquisition in the period of slow decline ; the first may have lost 40 per cent. of its value in the same time that the second has lost only 5 per cent.

We have thus found facts which are identical with those which Pavlov demonstrated concerning conditioned in-hibition, and to which we have called attention earlier.

[1] When spontaneous forgetting is studied, it is necessary to allow for the influence of these artificial processes of effacement. In the able pioneer studies of Ebbinghaus on the law of forgetting (1885), this source of error was not avoided. It modified the form of the initial process, hastening the appearance of the drop and accelerating it.

PART FOUR

INTELLECTUAL REACTIONS AND THE ELABORATION OF EXPERIENCE

Chapter I

THE ASSOCIATION PROCESS AND THE ACTION OF MEMORY

WE have spoken of the laws of mnemonic phenomena without considering any distinction between habit and memory. In current language, habit is reserved for motor learning. Progress in learning typewriting is a habit; the acquisition of a poem is an act of memory. But, in reciting verse, motor learning may, at least for some persons, be an essential part of the memory. There is no fundamental difference between the different modes of the mnemonic process.

Generally to-day all learning, all acquisitions which are perfected by repetition, are regarded as habits,[1] and memory is reserved for the recall of unique events which it is not possible to repeat, to pass through again. Thus Bergson distinguishes the memory of a piece of poetry which may be recited after a certain number of readings, and which is a habit, from the memory of one or another of the readings, the third or the fourth, which is pure memory.

There is nothing essential, however, in the distinction. The recitation is the result of motor reactions which are arranged in a certain manner, but can be produced by a

[1] The progress of learning implies a re-enforcement of chains of association which is shown by the acceleration and growth of precision and by the requirement of less effort (or less diffusion into parasitic acts which become eliminated).

series of visual or auditory recalls, as the reading is produced by one series of perceptions ; recitation can also follow a single perception if it covers a sufficiently short and impressive text.

There is an identity of mechanism in the recitation of a text and the reproduction by an artist of the head of a model, a visual image causing reactions of drawing, whether the latter be after a single perception or after repeated perceptions and successive sketches. Evidently reading implies that repetitions of the same text may be superimposed, through a second reading, a unique event, might be remembered, but only in the sense that there was a recall of the supplementary perceptions which have accompanied the perceptions of the text, and which were not the same for the different acts of repetition (an opening of the door, an impression of admiration, a feeling of weariness, a sudden noise, etc.).

But, so far as the consequences are concerned, there is no difference in nature between frequently repeated and unique, perceptive associations and there are all sorts of transitions. I attend a theatre and have a memory of it which has quite the character of a unique event ; if I return a second time, and especially if I am obliged professionally to follow all the successive presentations, the piece becomes an habitual memory ; but, in so far as I connect the different presentations to dates and incidents, each may be a unique memory in that part which has been different and not repeated. One of the incidents, if it is regularly reproduced, will become integrated in the habit memory and cease to be pure memory. Between memory founded on frequent associations of perceptions and that which is founded on a single association, there is the same difference as between the number *one* and various other numbers.

A memory always consists of the fixation of an associative connection, which permits a reaction to be reproduced whenever a given stimulus occurs. The reaction may be verbal when I pronounce a name on seeing a photograph, a reaction of recall when I picture a face to myself on hearing a name, or a drawing reaction if I sketch the outline of the face.

The mechanism of fixation is fundamentally the same as that which accounts for the origin of the conditioned reflex. But this is not equivalent to saying that, thanks to a knowledge of fundamental laws, it is possible to understand and predict the action of mnemonic processes like the action of conditioned reflexes. In an individual who is an organism, a unity, the mental processes form a tremendously complex mass in close mutual solidarity. The conditions for isolating a process, artificially realized in experimental psychology, are not found in life. All past experience, the whole system of tendencies and sentiments, intervenes at every moment in the course of any mnemonic process whatever.

We may ask why is a group of syllables more difficult for a well-informed individual to retain than a group of substantives in his language, a group of substantives more difficult than a verse of poetry? It is because the individual benefits from his previous acquisitions, from the memory of words which he has already acquired, from the known model of phrases, and because he is more interested in beautiful verse.

The utilization of what is already known in the acquisition of what is newly given is a normal process in the actual play of memory. There is an organization of perception which systematizes it, intellectualizes it, and integrates it with constructions prepared in advance. There is an organization of apprehension which permits a Poincaré to repeat eleven numbers after a single reading by noting the progressions and known relations among the numbers. There is an organization of mnemonic fixation which economizes effort by utilizing already familiar outlines for " comprehending," that is, for reducing the unknown to the known. Furthermore, as soon as the intellectualization occurs, varying extraordinarily as it does with individuals and with the nature of the material, complex factors intervene to mask the effects of elementary factors on which depend the mnemonic laws which we have noted. Interest, affective elements, may exercise an exceptionally favourable effect on the mnemonic fixation of a particular perception. It is for this reason that the memory of an event, even though unique, may—exceptionally, it is true—appear as solidly fixed as a memory based on many repetitions.[1] These memories of unique events are not, however, usually so firmly fixed as when the events are recalled or thought over again. This is because, if the external event no longer has the power to arouse the perceptions in the same context, the recall of this context becomes a mental event, which implies in its turn a mnemonic fixation that is stronger the more often the mental event is repeated.

In these repetitions, however, which are not strictly guided by the external phenomena, there are produced, under many influences, deformities and deviations which become fixed by repetition. The experimental study of testimony shows how general are these mistakes in the memory of an event, mistakes which are emphasized with time and with the repetition of the accounts of the event.[2]

In transmitting the account of an event from one person to another and then to a third, and so on, the addition of individual modifications, felt with the same certainty, leads to a recital which often has only a distant resemblance to the initial fact. The exaggeration of figures, for example, corresponds to a sentiment of astonishment which tends to justify them.

Again, in the recitation of a text learned by heart, there are analogous changes introduced solely by the fixating

[1] Whenever the emotion is too violent, it may, just as a trauma, have the contrary effect, since a perturbation of the organism reaching the nervous metabolism, interferes with the fixation of the memory of events which accompanied or preceded the affective shock. But in general the emotions have a very clear fixating influence, which is shown even among animals. A lizard which has been surprised by the violently disagreeable taste of a caterpillar avoids touching in any way another caterpillar resembling it.

[2] In successive accounts of the same dream, the change in form is especially pronounced, in the sense of a more coherent and more logical elaboration.

action of the repetitions, when it is repeated successively without reading it again.

Whenever the control of perceptive experience is no longer exercised, as when the physical or social surroundings have changed, the recall of places and people becomes decidedly inadequate. Whenever a person is confronted anew with the reality, as when he returns to a city which he left in childhood, he is surprised at the complete disagreement.

This is due to the simultaneous effect of the disappearance of the original memories and the mnemonic fixation of mental events caused by the attempts to recall the old memories, with the accompanying gaps and replacements. Thus it is that actual forgetting does not follow the simple law of the organic disappearance of associative bonds, which are revealed by their latent power to save a new effort of fixation. Moreover, the practical notion of forgetting is not concerned with the gradual disappearance of the impression, but with the diminution of the capacity, at a given moment, to utilize the memory.

We ask under what form this capacity shows itself. I see a person pass whose name I have known. If the name is not forgotten, the power to pronounce and write it is recalled. If I cannot think of the name at once I say that I have forgotten it, but I know very well that the memory has not entirely vanished. The proof is that, if a series of names are pronounced to me, I know that it is not any one of them. This is what Abramowski has called the " resistance of the forgotten."

I know that I will recognize the name, and, actually, when it is pronounced, I say, " that is it." The degree of forgetting is less than if the name is not even recognized.

Simple recognition is then a lower stage of the capacity to utilize memory.[1] Suppose that there is a painting which I recognize having seen ; I have a true memory of it only if I recall the artist and the museum where I have

---

[1] It is probable that the impression of recognition, or the feeling of familiarity, is connected with preliminaries of recall which are not carried through, not completely connected.

seen it. The localization of a memory is only the capacity to recall certain mnemonic connections with the occasion of the perception, and thus place it. It is the same as the capacity to recall the name of a friend when I see his face.

Practical utilization of a memory is essentially recall, the actualization of an associative bond.

The activity of memory is association, and association, putting mental content to work, is fundamentally mnemonic in nature.

Experimental researches on phenomena of association demonstrate the mnemonic bonds.[1] For example, the time which elapses between the perception of a word or of a picture and the word recalled, or associated (" association time "), is shorter the more frequently the two terms have been connected in perceptive experience, the stronger has become their mnemonic connection.

A certain community of environment and of education produces mnemonic relationships between words, so that the associative recall of one by the other is common and rapid. Mind-readers and prestidigitators utilize these habitual associations. It is thus that, when a person is asked to think very quickly of a colour and to write its name on a paper, one may claim to read his thought by declaring that the colour which he has written is red. About eight times out of ten it is this association which is spontaneously formed.

There is normally in most cases an individual emphasis, caused by a mental history which is different from that of other people.[2] The multiplicity of mnemonic connections causes a concurrence among the series of possible associations, of which one or another, depending upon the surrounding conditions, the time, etc., will be actually realized.

---

[1] The factors of association enumerated by William James—recency, frequency, vividness, and emotional affinity—are actually factors of mnemonic fixation, except the first, which implies less forgetting.

[2] In Rosanoff's studies of association in mental pathology, the main fact disclosed is that common associations are fewer among the insane, whose mental history is in fact abnormal.

It is the most simple primitive conception which regards mental activity as constituted by a linear chain of associations so that one chain is necessarily connected to another well defined chain. In mental individuality, in which there is a notably intimate solidarity, an associative recall is the resultant of a complex of factors, of feelings, of tendencies, of perceptions, of effects persisting after preceding activities, etc. The physical environment, the social milieu, the biological conditions all play their part. If a person is in the woods or in his study, if he faces an experimenter as a subject, is with an intimate friend or with a woman whom he is courting, if he is hungry or sleepy, etc., the same perceptions, the same words will not have in general the same power of recall.

When certain memories tend to be recalled, they do not always develop. They are inhibited or interfered with whenever an inconvenient image or troublesome idea faintly appears, of which we are ashamed or which at least we do not care to reveal. When there is an excessive retardation of the associative response called forth in experiments, it is supposed that there has been a struggle and that the perception aroused has awakened ideas and special feelings, called by the psychoanalysts a " complex," which the individual does not allow to be completed, to be expressed in behaviour, nor in mental activity.

Systematic investigation by paired associations, either controlled or free, the relations of words, images and ideas, has established certain categories of associative connection, which have shown that direct mnemonic relation was not always an adequate explanation of the recall.

Besides some acquired automatisms, pairs united in perceptive experience, terms are found to be called forth because they respond to a common feeling, or an analogous system of ideas, or because they imply similar sensory images (the assonance of certain words, for example). The predominance of affective, intellectual, or sensory and verbal associations, varies with the individual, the time, and the circumstances.

These associations, which form the thread of mental

activity, are nothing but the play of thought.   This rests entirely on the indispensable formation of mnemonic connections, on the acquisition of experience, but is not to be confounded with the action of memory.   In fact, thought implies an original elaboration of experience, and constitutes also a particular form of activity, an aspect of conduct, especially developed in our civilized societies, thanks to the utilization of a rich symbolism developed by many human generations.

Chapter II

THE ORGANIZATION OF SYMBOLISM

LANGUAGE AND THOUGHT

In experiments on the association of ideas, reference is made either to what is called free association of ideas—in which, on the appearance of a word or a picture, the subject says the first thing which comes to his mind or the whole chain of ideas which follow ; or to controlled association —in which the subject is required to respond to a word by its opposite, or by a word which has the same sound, or to submit to some other prescribed condition as directed.

But this opposition is only relative, since all association is directed which does not result solely from putting mnemonic automatisms in play. The same word may excite very different responses, and the predominance of one of these is due to directing factors, such as the perceptions, the feelings, the needs, etc.

Under ordinary circumstances, the associative play of thought responds to the exigencies of life, to the necessities of continuous adaptation to the physical surroundings and to the social background. It is an instrument of action. Thought has been well called " controlled association."

Thought, however, is not entirely free from its essentially mnemonic origin. It is organization of experience, but it cannot exist except in so far as associative bonds assure the acquisition of experience. The primitive form of experience which permits the organism to fortify itself against certain menacing influences, or to prepare in advance for certain conquests, rests upon the anticipation which results from the action of the conditioned reflex and is translated into all forms of conduct. The sight of delicious fruit suffices to release the salivary reflex which was connected at first only with the taste of the fruit; it thus suffices to awaken the perception which anticipates the agreeable taste, and to direct the acts which will provide for renewing the desired experience.

A simple fragment of a complex situation, in connection with which it has often been found, is sufficient to arouse the conduct which is suited to this situation. This is what characterizes perception, which, though an elementary one, is nevertheless an act of thought.

If two different situations have certain common features, when a person becomes accustomed to one of them he will act in the same manner in the presence of the other, under the influence of the common fragmentary experience. He will choose, for eating, fruit of the same form and colour as that which he knows has an agreeable taste. This is the foundation of attitudes and thoughts of analogy which play a very considerable role in the life of animals and man.

On the other hand, if a person is deceived, this will produce, in connection with any characteristic, a conditioned inhibition, an arrest of a similar tendency. Thus experience becomes complicated and blended as we adapt ourselves to new circumstances in the course of " trial and error," of groping behaviour.

At the same time the capacity for individual progress, for personal acquisition of experience, is necessarily very limited. Social organization, thanks to the development of language, permits new generations of humanity to benefit from the gropings, from the trials and errors of many generations which have disappeared.

Language represents a systematization of the fundamental process of symbolism. This is not of social origin, but results from the action of the same laws of individual thought which cause analogous attitudes. Even perception is symbolic, in so far as a sensory excitant, selected from a group, takes on a significant value, and, as a substitute for this group, is aroused in place of it, releasing appropriate acts. The noise of a spoon in a bowl becomes for a young child the symbol of his dinner, the barking of a dog is the symbol of an animal which barks, and, by analogous extension, the widespread character of which we have noted, the symbol is formed for different animals. In the same way, when pronouncing " wa-wa " significantly, the baby will express quite a wide range of possible experiences, in the form of a real symbolic reaction.

Vocal expressions, which furnish the means of affecting other beings (cries to alarm, to call, or to arouse pity) easily take on symbolic significance. Their systematic development constitutes language. In a social group this is transmitted by education to new individuals in the group. The vocal expressions, in all their flexible variety, are practised by children ; and association with perceptive experiences causes their meaning and function to be progressively learned, through the double movement of association by analogy which extends the usage of terms, and of conditioned inhibition which restricts and adapts the usage, in the course of the trials and errors of mental life.

In our Mediterranean civilizations language has taken a more and more dominating place. It has developed, in a complex hierarchy, symbols of symbols, or conceptual symbols, each, by a wide extension, designating a category symbolic terms of more limited signification. In such circumstances verbal conduct has often arrived at a condition of being sufficient unto itself. An expression becomes an act which is no longer presented as a means, but constitutes an end—discourse, poetry, romance, or simply play of words. In the education of children the symbolic character of words has come to be neglected. It is forgotten to attach to a perceptual content—the essential basis of the whole verbal edifice—the vocal or written expressions, learned for their own sakes.

This development of verbalism in our civilizations, which have, thanks to it, been able to erect a world system of high utilitarian value, has, in practice, brought about a real identification of thought and language.

The convenient employment of symbolic substitutes for

all perceptive experiences becomes so general that most
educated individuals retain, recall, foresee and prepare for
all experience, for all activity, through the use of verbal
forms exclusively. Furthermore, collective education
tends to compel thought to conform constantly to the
framework of grammatical constructions, to the coherence
of logical conceptual schemes, in spite of affective influences and sensory contingencies. Often, it is true,
thought escapes from this rigid framework. It is the rule,
however, to stamp out irregularities, or to conceal
them as moral faults, a rule against which certain
modernistic literary schools are to-day in revolt.

It is in the dream, in the abandonment accompanying
reverie, such as the Freudian practice of psycho-analysis
seeks to produce, that thought escapes from the constraint
of social logic, even when preserving a verbal character.
But in the successive accounts of an incoherent dream a
progressive change in form occurs in the direction of
logical reconstruction, conforming to a framework of
thought controlled by a whole intellectualistic civilization
(Foucault).

Thought should be verbal in order that it may be
communicated, and it is scarcely considered thought until
it is communicable in nature. Socialized man is no longer
an organism capable of withdrawing itself from affairs,
and becoming isolated in the midst of a hostile nature.
Thought forms part of a common heritage from which man
borrows and to which he contributes. He is obliged to
submit to its verbal structure.

The experimental study of the thought of civilized
adults submitted to such collective constraint cannot,
therefore, fail to show a rather uniform content. When
thinking in words, one person may believe that he
only hears them or tends to say them ; another may
sometimes recall a written representation of them ; but
such individual differences are of little consequence. But
are the words which are never lacking among
normal people adequate or must they be supplemented by
different elements ? The different theories of thought

answer this question in many ways, relying upon experimental results obtained, in pursuance of a method due to Binet, by various investigators, in particular by Marbe, Bühler, and the Würzburg School. These results were obtained by questioning the subjects who were to think about the nature of thought, and by making them describe the processes with which they had to become intimately acquainted. But the conclusions are unfortunately impregnated with theory for the very reason that they must be expressed in the words provided and must conform to a verbal framework. Discussion of the reality and nature of " imageless thought " has therefore elicited quite contradictory facts in connection with the different schools—if such introspective results can really be called facts.

When it is necessary to record, without theoretical preconceptions, any verbal reactions rendering explicit the course of a thought, it is quite apparent that, with individual differences, the fundamental elements are verbal representations. These are supplemented at times—especially when the thought is not directed with too much haste towards an interesting outcome, or does not follow too quickly the guidance of the reading matter—by various perceptive representations, very unequal in development, of a sensory nature and predominantly auditory or visual among most individuals.

The quicker the thought the less the concrete support of these representations is in evidence, the more it remains in the sphere of abstract symbolisms. But these symbolisms always fall back on representations. Are there no cases, no moments, when this support fails to bridge the two verbal banks of stream of thought, definite, though obviously brief ?

I read a phrase and I comprehend it. Comprehension appears as an act of thought. When required to express a judgment, I approve it and think it is correct, or I deny it because it is false ; I recognize and appreciate the relation of terms, the hierarchy of the two concepts. In what form are these characteristic operations of thought

clothed ? They are expressed in words, as " I comprehend," " I know," " It is true," " It is false," etc.
These are expressive reactions which are sometimes occur
in the form of silent representations. But it is quite
apparent that it is possible to comprehend without
speaking, without saying " I comprehend." What, then,
is comprehension ? To comprehend is in reality to adopt
an adequate attitude, whether this be a mental attitude
or an objective one.

If, in a meeting, someone starts to make disagreeable
remarks against which I am prepared to protest, and I
am signalled that the person is mentally unbalanced ; if
I comprehend the signal, I will abstain from speaking and
will adopt an indulgent attitude. My whole manner in
relation to the person concerned will be modified.

Comprehending an argument, which changes an opinion
of mine, consists in modifying, as a result, a system of
ideas.

But, if the comprehension has objective significance in
the course of the processes of thought, which end in
definite results of more or less general bearing and
relatively complete external expression, there is in addition
the *knowledge* which I have, in comprehension. At every
moment I am informed of the steps in my thought, just as
sensations let me know of the status of the execution of a
movement or an action.

It is really the nature of this knowledge, of this information, which constitutes the true problem for those
who theorize about thought. It has often been admitted
that it is by sensations of a kinæsthetic order, due to
characteristic attitudes which we never fail to take in
relation to various judgments and various processes of
thought, that we gain our information. And, in
point of fact, objective examination shows that the
attitudes are different if a person comprehends or not, if
he approves or objects, if he recognizes something as
familiar or is astonished by it.

But do these attitudes constitute—not the thought,
evidently, although this has been claimed—the support
for the knowledge of our thought, or are they really

secondary matters, which have a significance, a symbolic value, but which might disappear without anything changing ?   It is the same problem which has occurred to theorists regarding the emotions (the knowledge of the emotion), regarding attention (the knowledge of our state of attention), etc.

Or, again, are we here concerned with feelings, agreeable or disagreeable, of facility, of immediate recall, of decision, of something out of place, etc., which, in the course of the actual steps of the thought, permit us to say, to make known, the place reached by the work of the mind, as if a special reaction were able to furnish a kind of instantaneous view of the progress of the operation ?

These feelings certainly exist and have a regulative role ; but whether they are reducible to sensations or not, cannot be affirmed with certainty.   This is not, moreover, of essential importance for the real problem, for that is concerned not with the mechanism of reflection about thought, but with the mechanism of thought itself.

Chapter III

CREATIVE THOUGHT AND THE ECONOMY OF EXPERIENCE

An important function of the symbolism of thought is the condensation of experience. This permits the benefit of a multitude of acquired results to be secured by economizing memory. Certain words take the place of a mass of perceptive representations. The key to their symbolism once being known, such words can be substituted, from one person or from one generation to another, for the acquisition of most of the inter-related representations. This condensation of experience saves time both for the individual and the group.

The development of symbolism has also brought with it, through education and perhaps through heredity, the progressive atrophy of the capacity to recall concrete images which may be projected with almost the force and of hallucinations. This capacity is no longer encountered except among certain children, according to Jaensch, who has called these results " eidetic " images.

The educational tendency to replace realistic images by more manageable abstract outlines, especially for collective usage, is universal—except among painters or musicians, whose thoughts are still based on concrete visual or auditory images and who express themselves in society by painting or by instrumental execution aided by the symbolism of musical notation. For many men the tendency is carried into their dreams, verbalism extending throughout their mental life, while images vivid and rich enough to recall the actual perceptions are quite exceptional. Moreover, when a person thinks that he has images, the analysis shows that they are singularly schematic. Abstract expression is substituted for the purely concrete.

In place of a storehouse of facts, thanks to a verbal law, to a rule of symbolism, we learn how to reconstruct them. The sciences permit this to be done correctly with increasing simplicity, by embracing under the most economical form the greatest number of results.

There is another important function of thought, the very formal framework of which has been furnished us by collective elaboration. This is logical reasoning, which brings about an economy, not of memories of acquired experience, but in the acquisition of experience itself. Thought permits us to avoid groping, trial and error responses which are present in the modes of adaptation of nearly all organisms.

As Mach well observed, thought, in the activity of reasoning, is above all an imaginative experience.

By means of reasoning, remarks Rignano, we can state with certainty that, in a great city like London, it is possible to find two individuals with the same number of hairs on their heads. This follows from the fact that the number of inhabitants is greater than the maximum number of hairs which it is possible for a single individual to have. All the inhabitants may be imagined ranked according to the number of their hairs. We are thus assured that in some ranks it will be necessary to include more than one individual.

The experiment, which it would not be exactly easy to carry through, is thus rendered unnecessary.

Experiments have been made on numerous animals and on children of various ages, to determine in what cases, when facing a difficulty, a new situation requiring an adaptation, the solution, if it is found at all, will be obtained only by grouping, by trials made at random, and in what cases, on the contrary, it will be made by a systematic act of thought.

Boutan states, for example, that an anthropoid ape, like the gibbon, will succeed in opening a box containing something good to eat, and held closed by an unfamiliar

K

mechanism, only by continued trials pursued at random. A young child, not yet able to speak, proceeds in exactly the same way. But children a little older when placed in front of the box to be opened, reflect, hunt for relations of cause and effect, direct their trials—which at first cannot be entirely avoided—and, the success obtained, know why, so that they do not begin again by making the errors in case of a new test. The ape, on the contrary, having succeeded in opening the box by chance, will continue to try other movements, and the tendency to the effective action will be selectively re-enforced by a frequently repeated association between a certain movement and the prize of the food.

In observing thus the failure of an infant which did not speak and an anthropoid which never speaks, it is a temptation to think that only the logical tool due to society permits thought to be substituted for empirical groping. Language would then be the necessary instrument of thought.

But other more highly evolved anthropoid apes, for example, the chimpanzee, whose rudimentary language is far from being a social tool, are capable of directed trials, of mental inventions which economize the gropings. This has been established by various systematic investigations, the most convincing of which is due to Köhler.

Mental anticipation exists then, although in a rudimentary form, with the chimpanzee. It becomes the rule when, with language and logical habits, civilized man acquires a reliable instrument of knowledge and action.

Education in our European civilization[1] carries with it prescriptions for the solution of problems, for adaptation to the difficulties of physical and social life. In order that the engineer may construct a bridge or the merchant fix

[1] The instrument of thought is really quite different in oriental civilizations. It is directed more towards internal satisfaction than towards subduing nature, more penetrated with mystic feeling than preoccupied with logical understanding. For such civilizations language is more a means of social action, for the communication of sentiments and æsthetic expression than for intellectual objective systematization.

his prices, it is only necessary to follow well-defined rules of algebraic or arithmetic thought, in order to attain certain results.

The difficulty in attacking a new problem is always in putting it into an equation, at least in correctly stating it, in appreciating the essential principles and rules which apply to it.

In studying how a person proceeds in the face of a relatively new problem, it is observed that he returns to the primitive and eternal biological method, that of trial and error. It is by groping, during which a point of provisional departure is adopted, a procedure is attempted, that results are attained. Though the trials may be systematic enough for the most part, there will also be a considerable lack of co-ordination when we rely on chance inspiration. But the influence of principles of thought can be seen in the registration of the negative result of certain attempts. From the defeat itself, lessons are drawn for the future.

In this essential function of thought, which, in the course of its gropings comes to avoid the delays and the dangers of the experience lived through, and which is not blocked by material impossibilities, successive points of vantage may be distinguished. First is the location of the problem, the comprehension of the question, the delimitation of the difficulty to be solved ; second is the invention of a solution ; and third, the critical verification of the value of the imagined solution.

It is at the second point especially that thought is truly creative. But creation is seen to rest on extensions by analogy, on the employment of learned procedures. Very rarely is there true invention, unforeseeable, escaping experimental investigation. In fact the action of thought may lead in a certain measure to representative or conceptual imaginings of a new character.[1] But if neither

[1] Besides the necessities of life, which impose on thought more or less difficult questions, whenever the ease and security of existence permits the luxury of free imagination, the feelings come to exercise on mental activity a directing influence, relatively co-ordinated, extending to the lucubrations of the dream and even to the amorous poetry of the adolescent at the crisis of puberty.

science nor art is able to utilize these results they are eliminated by the individual or by society, which relegates both them and their authors to the asylums.

What appears from time to time to be unique in character, is the invention which leads to some large and fruitful conception or some new form of art. The mental genesis of such inventions, in which the chance of certain contacts of facts or ideas often plays an essential role, is difficult to trace, since it is essentially what eludes experimental investigation.

But, if the great and celebrated inventions are compared with the modest work of the mind bent on imagining the solution of some unaccustomed problem, as numerous transitions give us the right to do, it is possible by extrapolation, as the complexity increases, to extend to the former the mental determinism shown in the latter.

PART FIVE

THE LEVELS OF ACTIVITY AND THE UTILIZATION OF EXPERIENCE

Chapter I

THE DEGREES OF MENTAL EFFICIENCY AND THE NOTION OF ATTENTION

An individual, under stimulation, is able to take different attitudes corresponding to the external excitants. A child who sees a pretty coloured butterfly, tries to catch it as it flies by. If a toad jumps near him, he avoids it with disgust. If he sees the grass move just beside him, he stops and tries to discover what caused the movement, ready to flee if it is a snake, or, if it is a wounded bird, prompt to pick it up.

These three attitudes are attitudes of interest. The first two are adapted to the nature of the object, and are called perceptive. The third, called pre-perceptive,[1] is an endeavour to become acquainted with an object and to prepare an adapted response. All three represent definite and unified orientation of behaviour. They

[1] The perceptive interest is awakened by a certain correspondence between the nature of the object perceived and the appropriate tendencies of the individual and corresponds to their actual strength. The sight of food awakens an interest which varies with the degree of hunger and disappears with it. The pre-perceptive interest is awakened by a change, especially by a sudden and quick movement (an object which will arouse reflex visual attention) and by intense and unexpected stimuli. The perceptive adaptation follows, along with a response of more complete exploration, of acquisition of knowledge (corresponding to curiosity). Then comes utilization or flight, or finally an attitude of disinterest, neglecting the object or phenomenon, turning away from it, or regarding it as of no further use.

constitute the reaction of " attention." Attention is, as McDougall[1] has well described it, a notion which expresses the existence of an interest and of a corresponding orientation of the activity and of the attitudes. This orientation is definite and unified in the sense that the entire organism is subordinated to the direction imposed by the fundamental interest.

It is this general unification of activity, expressing the individualizaiton of the organism, which is characteristic and which is called attention, a term which does not refer to any defined and self-acting process.

If the child, having seen the grass move near him, considers that it was merely the effect of a gust of wind, he will not be interested in it (perceptive reaction of disinterest) ; that is to say, he will cease to pay attention, to occupy himself with it, to subordinate his conduct to this negligible motion ; and he will direct his activity in another way, according to his dominant interest. For example, he will pick a flower or chase a bee.

If any interest does not manifest itself, if any direction does not solicit activity, then activity will cease, and the organism fall into a state of lassitude which may produce the process of sleep. This involves an abolition of all adaptive behaviour, of the entire perceptive process.[2] until a lively enough stimulus excites interest anew[3] and brings about a resumption of oriented activity which can be described as an awakening of attention.

The process of attention is, then, a unified orientation of behaviour. It implies a canalization of the phenomena of static or dynamic activity in a certain direction, and the arrest of activity in every other possible direction ; an

---

[1] " Interest," says he, " is latent attention, and attention is interest in action." (*An Outline of Psychology*, 1923, p. 277.)

[2] Sleep involves an active process of the inhibition of the sensori-motor activities. It is not only the absence of an adapted activity and of orientation of behaviour which characterizes sleep, but the opposition to the adaptation of activity, to oriented behaviour.

[3] Under the influence of general inhibition which characterizes sleep, these tendencies of interest are unequally repressed. They preserve, according to their strength a relatively great susceptibility to being awakened. A mother is aroused by the feeble cry of her infant, while a much more violent noise in the street will not attract her attention and interrupt her sleep.

inhibition of all forms of behaviour which do not accord with the dominant orientation.

An elementary phenomenon of attention is furnished by the behaviour of an inferior organism in which the individuality is incompletely established, the starfish. In the communal activity of the starfish one of the five arms becomes predominant, which makes it the director commanding the general movement of the star. At a time when the starfish is moving, if, from behind it, an odorous pear is brought near one of the arms, the movement will be inhibited, and the arm excited by the odour will at once start to go towards the pear. The others will follow it and subordinate their movements to it. There is thus produced, under the influence of the stimulus and the reaction of perceptive interest which it has engendered, a process of orientation of behaviour with the inhibition of other activities, a process of attention.[1]

The greater the stimulation, the greater will be the reaction of attention, that is to say, the more intense will be the inhibition and the more marked the orientation under the influence of this stimulation. The change of behaviour will be more rapid, the movement more prompt and more precise ; the efficiency will be increased. We have here all the essential characteristics of the process of attention and of its levels, which represent the levels of efficiency of behaviour.

These characteristics are encountered in a certain measure in the functioning of the infra-cortical nerve centres in man and the other mammals. The individuality of the organism implies a co-ordination of automatic activities and reflexes. This requires re-enforcements and inhibitions electively distributed. The precision in this co-ordinated distribution of re-enforced or restricted actions, and the energy of these actions, may show various

---

[1] This process is correlative to the development of the nerve centres of co-ordination, the role of which is properly to assure the unity of the individual, the individuality of conduct. By destroying the central nerve ring of the starfish, or cutting the connections of the arms with these centres, we can abolish co-ordination and the processes of unification which are exercised by elective re-enforcement and inhibition, that is to say, the process of attention, in the starfish.

degrees. The neurologist Head has called these the degrees of " vigilance."[1]

But it is above all in the functioning of the superior centres, regulating the mental processes, that is to say, in the unified behaviour, that the vigilance, namely, the attention, has the greatest importance and manifests itself more obviously.

The intensity of attention, representing the level of efficiency for one activity, directed in a certain way, is a function of the interest involved, the natural and direct interest or the secondary interest.[2] In other words the intensity of attention is a function (a) of the magnitude of affective factor orienting behaviour, which frees energies, either of release or of arrest ; and (b) of the disposable quantity of these energies, which are distributed in the form of static or dynamic forces and in the form of more or less numerous inhibitions.   These activities and inhibitions in the case of thought are exclusively associative in nature.

In the case of great fatigue, after strong emotions or prolonged insomnia, the capacity of attention—the affective value of the stimulus remaining constant for the individual—will be notably diminished, because the disposable energies are at a minimum.

Certain individuals have less capacity of attention than others, either on account of the feebleness of their interests or on account of the small amount of energy they have available.   The latter condition is very noticeable among " neurasthenics."

For an equal affective force, the efficiency thus depends upon the energy disposable ; for equal energies, the

[1] A de-cerebrate mammal, dog or cat for example, and also a " spinal" cat, that is to say, one in which the medulla alone still controls the processes of activity, is susceptible to very unequal levels of efficiency depending upon its physiological state, corresponding to the functional vitality of its nerve centres, as if the level of attention varied in the execution of automatic activities or reflexes.

[2] According to the nature of the interest, one speaks of " spontaneous" (automatic) attention and " voluntary " attention ; but it is a distinction which can be extended to all the modes of activity, of behaviour, and which we shall examine in connection with the notion of " will." It has no special bearing upon the process of attention as such.

efficiency depends upon the interest, upon the affective force of the stimulus. It increases with the latter up to a certain optimum, beyond which the emotional perturbation with its diffusion of inco-ordinations will tend to diminish the efficiency.

The process of attention appears then to be very complex ; it seems to be the resultant of multiple factors, transferring themselves under the form of greater or less efficiency in the one definite direction of co-ordinated activity of the organism.[1]

Furthermore, the notion of the measurement of attention, which ranks among the foremost preoccupations of experimental psychology and which psychotechnology has borrowed, must appear in a form very different from that which would be implied by the concept of a simple function—as a sort of faculty of attention. In reality one measures only efficiencies. From the practical point of view this is of incontestable importance. To take account of the capacity for efficiency in one or another sort of activity, is, in effect, to allow the individuals in any kind of organization to be better utilized.[2]

These efficiencies are measured from points of view

---

[1] The automatic activities are free, in their execution, from the higher individual co-ordination, which controls their release. Moreover, the attention does not augment the efficiency of these activities ; but, on the contrary, diminishes and disturbs their accomplishment, as when one raises the question how to breathe or to walk or to keep one's balance. This fact is well symbolized in an Indian legend according to which the centipede, asking his hundred feet to tell him the order in which he advances them, becomes so confused that he is unable to walk at all.

" When asked which leg went after which,
He lay distraught within the ditch,
Considering how to go."

[2] It is possible to " test " attention by discovering the subject's efficiency in crossing out certain letters in a text (taking account of the errors and omissions), or dotting with a pencil small circles which move before the subject, to recognize objects from incomplete pictures, etc. The increase in the apparent intensity of a sensation, which certain authors claim to trace to greater clearness, furnishes also an evaluation of the degree of attention, especially in the form of lowering the threshold. A stimulus which starts a sensorial process which is too weak to pass over into a perception of the impression integrated in behaviour, will pass this threshold under the influence of the appropriate perceptive orientation, of an effort of sensorial attention.

which may differ considerably since they involve, in the execution of a prescribed activity, both absolute magnitudes and speeds. A given task may be performed more or less well, more or less quickly. The final assessment must take account both of perfection and of rapidity of execution, with relative values susceptible of considerable variation. The rapidity in certain cases is of great importance, and in others almost negligible.

The precision or strength of certain movements, the exactness of certain choices or of certain calculations made, the reasonableness of conclusions, the precision of percepts or concepts, the intensity of sensorial impressions, represent some of the measurable modes in absolute efficiency. Speed of perception, speed of movement, speed of calculation or of thought, constitute other measurable modes of efficiency relative to time.[1]

By experiment we study—in the absolute accomplishment and in the speed of execution of a task—the efficiency of an individual at a given moment for a prescribed action ; that is to say, under defined conditions of a strictly social character implying a particular kind of interest.

For the same prescribed action not only the relative efficiency of individuals may be compared, and this is legitimate and fruitful ; but the efficiency of the same individual may be compared under varied conditions. Thus one estimates mental fatigue by the diminution of this efficiency ; one examines the effect—exciting or depressing—of different toxic substances or of various

[1] Attention may be studied by the " tapping test," which consists of hitting a strip of paper with a pencil in the most rapid rhythm possible; by the time of reaction (the interval between the production of a stimulus and the movement arranged for—simple reaction time ; between the production of different stimuli and given movements corresponding each time to the nature of the stimulus—discriminative reaction time with choice) ; by the measurement of the latency of perceptions (seeking the difference in time between two heterogeneous stimuli, a noise and a light stimulus for example, such that the stimulus towards which the attention is directed will yet appear simultaneously produced) ; and by the speed of (perceptions, tachistoscopic experiments determining the minimum time of presentation of an object compatible with exact perception).

influences of the surroundings[1] according to the increase or diminution of efficiency, etc.

Certain characteristics of efficiency especially lend themselves to fruitful researches ; in particular, its stability in time, its plasticity, and its extent, depending upon the multiplicity and complexity of the tasks performed simultaneously.

In a continuous activity, it is found that the efficiency does not remain constant, but presents spontaneous oscillations, which are shown in the speed of perceptions or of movements, in the strength or precision of acts, etc. These oscillations are rendered particularly evident when, in the course of perceptive attention, one observes a sensorial impression under the action of an uninterrupted stimulus.   If the intensity of the stimulus is near the threshold, the impression disappears and reappears periodically.   This may be observed, for example, for the tick of a watch placed at the farthest distance it can be heard, for the appearance of a shadow so feeble as to be only just distinguished, etc.

The period of these spontaneous oscillations, of a physiological order[2] is from 3 to 10 seconds.   They are not necessarily connected with apparent organic rhythms like the respiratory rhythm or the vaso-motor rhythm, produced by successive peripheral waves of vaso-dilation and of vaso-constriction.   At times external signs are observed (Pillsbury) of oscillations which are weaker and of shorter period, about a fifth of a second.

These oscillations are normal and differ relatively little from one individual to another.   But the stability of the efficiency depends above all on the stability of the interest, in the observance of directions, in the definite orientation

[1] For example, there is often an increase in efficiency through the factor of imitation, the presence of an audience, the presence of experimenters of the opposite sex, etc. ; the tonic influence is noted for certain general stimuli, for example, of light, showing the value of adequate illumination ; comparisons are made for the hours of the day, the days of the week, the seasons, meteorological conditions, etc.

[2] In following the oscillations of the apparent intensity of the perception of an electric stimulus of the skin and the reflex response of the winking of the eyelid to this stimulus, it is possible to determine (Martin) that they are entirely superimposed.

of the activity.   Submitting to diverse stimuli of external or associative origin, which tend to divert the interest or monopolize activity, an individual with a definite task resists these disturbing influences which the experimenter himself has introduced in order to measure their effects. What is the strength of the subject's resistance ?[1]   That may be determined from the continuous record of efficiency in making calculations, in crossing out letters, or in the times of reaction, etc., etc.

On the other hand, by changing the task at a given signal many times in succession, and by comparing the efficiency attained in each of these tasks, when combined from the successive periods, to that which is attained in an equal uninterrupted time for each, we measure the plasticity, the adaptive flexibility of the effort of attention during these changes in the orientation of the activity.

Similarly, if a person must perform several simultaneous tasks (for example, cross out letters in a text and count at the same time the beats of a metronome), what will happen to the efficiency in the execution of both tasks together, compared to the efficiency (always greater) in the execution of each task separately ?

It is found that those individuals who were most competent to undertake several tasks at a time also those who could change most easily and quickly the general orientation of their activity and who had the most suppleness of attention (quick and alert type).

In reality the attention, that is to say the orientation of the activity of an individual, is always unique at any particular moment ; but, by rapid changes, the attentive activity may be devoted to one task and another alternately for very short periods in such a way that the execution of the tasks may appear simultaneous. This is especially notable when one has command of the rhythm of a piece of work, in dotting, for example, letters which pass behind a window while counting rhythmical sounds.

[1] In studying the action of certain sensorial distractions there has sometimes been found, in certain individuals, an increase in efficiency. The necessity of resistance produces an increase in the effort of attention sufficient to rise above the earlier level of efficiency.

Various methods have shown that the change of orientation occurs very rapidly, in two or three tenths of a second,[1] and so in the course of a second one is able to return very nearly twice to each of two tasks executed at the same time.

The attention is sometimes appreciated, not in its direct and logical effects, that is to say at the level of efficiency ; but in its ordinary concomitants, in what is called its expression. There is thus a " physiognomy " of the attentive individual. It shows in the selective contraction of certain muscles of the face[2] and varies slightly according to the orientation of the attention, depending, for example, upon whether it is more visual or more auditory.

In the effort of attention there are some physiological modifications which tend simply to a diffusion of energy,[3] and which bring about useless increases in the tonic contractions of different muscles, and there are some adaptive modifications tending to favour the desired activity and to block disturbances.[4]

For example, the fixation of the eyes and the accommodation of vision to a convenient distance are related especially to visual attention ; the attitude of the head,

[1] Wundt recognized likewise that a tenth of a second was sufficient. To realize a maximum effort of attention it is always necessary to allow about one or two seconds. For this reason the time of reaction to a given stimulus is shortest when the interval between the warning signal and the stimulus is from 1 to 2 seconds, a little more for a visual stimulus, requiring fixation of the eyes, than for an auditory stimulus.

[2] Among the blind the attentive expression of the face is generally not noticeable. This indicates the predominance of the fixation of the eyes in the attentive expression of a normal person.

[3] Under the influence of effort, even when directed in a well defined way, the nervous influx overflows in numerous motor pathways, diffusing more widely as the effort increases. This indicates a greater expenditure of energy, as, for example, when the organism struggles against fatigue. There is an overflow into the autonomic system causing certain modifications of the rhythm of the heart (which is accelerated), of the respiration, etc. The phenomena of cerebral vaso-dilation, accompanied generally by peripheral vaso-constriction, indicate increased cerebral activity.

[4] General immobility, fixation of the eyes on a region of the visual field where nothing is happening, with relaxation of the accommodation of the lenses, also holding the breath for a time, all contribute to avoiding disturbances coming from tactual and kinæsthetic impressions or from vision (without shutting the eyes which is in general depressive). The distractions from sounds (the breathing and movements of the body being noisy) are likewise avoided.

turning one ear towards the probable region of the expected sound, and the accommodation of the tympanum, correspond to auditory attention ; the tension of the muscles of the limbs and the flexion of the body, with a forward displacement of the centre of gravity, are related to the motor attention of a runner about to start.

In the last case there is a special motor type of attention, in the first two a sensory type ;[1] but there are also some purely intellectual types of meditative attention in which there occurs a general inhibition of the perceptive processes and of adaptive motor reactions. The latter are often replaced by automatisms, which are usually inhibited, but are then freed by an exclusively mental orientation of the activity of the individual.

When introspective psychology, which may be deceived by the mirage of reflection, has asked what attention is, it has very naturally expected to find that everyone, when he gave himself up to an introspective task which had been assigned to him, could observe that he was attentive. Such psychology has been preoccupied with defining the criteria of this self-knowledge of the attention. What it has found was only the impressions of effort coming from muscular tensions increased by the diffusion of the nervous impulse which had been freed in excessive quantities.

The theories of attention known as " peripheral " explain the feeling of being attentive, confounded with the attentive process itself, by the cardiac, vascular, respiratory, muscular and other modifications, the perception of which constitutes the feeling in question.

We know, however, that it is necessary not to confound processes and the knowledge that we may have of them. These are distinct problems. Our internal perceptions, like our external perceptions, may be based on signs of a very varied nature.

---

[1] In meeting the same sensori-motor task, the attentive attitude may be more sensory or more motor : For example, in the task of reacting to a stimulus as quickly as possible (experiments with the time of reaction) there are some individuals who prepare for the perception of the stimulus and others for the reactional movement. The latter permits a more rapid reaction, but causes more errors if it is necessary to discriminate among several stimuli.

Chapter II

ACTIVITY AND WORK

INCITEMENT AND FATIGUE

The study of the efficiency of an activity corresponds to the problem of attention, but the different modes of activity lead to studies which are no longer concerned with general efficiency except in a secondary way.

The two principal forms of activity are the sensori-motor and the mental, while in transition from one to the other there are numerous forms of mixed activity, among which the verbal holds an important place.

Mental activity ends in an affirmation (the solution of a problem, a logical deduction, an imaginative construction, the result of a calculation, etc.), after a series of operations of thought conforming to a general control, which may be imposed as directions by an experimenter.

Sensori-motor activity responds to tasks of quite varied complexity, and occupying very different places in a hierarchy. To make dots on a paper, to strike out all the letters in a text, or certain letters, or certain groups of letters, and finally to cancel words having certain letters in common, or having a certain common meaning, all imply, indeed, common sensori-motor mechanisms, but involving more and more complex mental operations, interposed between the impressions and the movements, the perceptual reaction taking place at a constantly rising level.

These are activities of the kind that may be observed, when attention is studied, by considering their precision, their correctness, and their speed.

Moreover, it is possible to examine—by supposing the same general level of efficiency—the effects on actual efficiency in a particular activity, brought about by a change in the conditions of this activity.

It is established, for example, that the speed with which a task is accomplished is in inverse relation to its complexity and direct relation to its familiarity, and that the precision tends to vary in inverse relation to the speed, but increases also with the familiarity of the task. These facts conform to the results of studies made from the point of view of memory and learning, of progress as a function of repetition.[1]

In the increase of precision and speed of activities in relation to their familiarity, it is observed that a part of this increase is due to general modifications of behaviour. and is shown for similar tasks carried out in analogous fashion ; but most of it is connected with modifications which are strictly limited to the systems of activity concerned.

After having distributed cards many times in a certain order, this action will be performed correctly in shorter and shorter time. If other cards are to be classified, the initial time will be less than if there had been no practice of this kind, but much longer than to carry out the habitual classification.

Learning to write readily with the right hand facilitates the acquisition of writing with the other hand, but it does not make this acquisition unnecessary. This is natural because of the asymmetry in the activity of the two hands in man.[2]

The acquired co-ordination of our movements agrees with the normal disposition of the ocular images on the retinas ; a change in their arrangement produces an

[1] This progress is at first rapid, then more and more slow. It is, perhaps, represented by a branch of the hyperbola (Foucault's Law of Exercise).

[2] There is in a child a spontaneous tendency to help itself with one of its hands, which as a result has more exercise and acquires more training through this practice, and also more strength. In 93% of the cases the preferred hand is the right, in 7% the left.

Among adults the force of contraction of the predominating hand (at least of the right hand when that is predominant), as measured by the dynamometer, is about 10% greater than that of the other hand. The differences are less marked among children than among adults, among women than among men, among peasants and manual workers (who use both hands more) than among intellectuals.

immediate inco-ordination. To verify this it is sufficient to try to trace around a five-pointed star while looking at the design of the star and the hand as reflected in a mirror. A real " apraxia," an incapacity to carry out correctly simple acts and habits, is thus experimentally brought about.[1]

When the time of reaction is measured, the time consumed is found to vary with the kind of response. For physiological causes a response of the leg will be slower than a response of the arm or the mouth. Furthermore, among the reactions of the arm, natural and spontaneous reactions will be carried out more quickly than conventional reactions. The latter are themselves more slow, the more artificial they are, the more rarely they occur in normal life.[2]

In activities of imposed rhythm, the precision of the rhythm will be obtained more easily as it coincides better, for the individual undertaking the task, with his own rhythmical tendency.[3]

Large individual differences in efficiency are encountered in complex forms of activities, because these activities are unequally familiar (language, singing, etc.). Certain of

[1] If certain activities, that of shaving, for example, are normally carried out with the use of a mirror, apraxia will be produced by obtaining the normal ocular images by the use of two mirrors.

[2] The reaction time includes : 1. The latent time required to start the sensory apparatus, a time which for a stimulus near the threshold may be very long, reaching and even exceeding a second, but decreasing very rapidly until it becomes negligible as the intensity of the stimulus increases. 2. The time of transmission of the centripetal and centrifugal nerve impulse. 3. The time of the perceptive order for the reaction, which is very variable, is the longest, and the reduction of it indicates the growth in efficiency. 4. Finally, the retardation of the muscular contraction. This last retardation varies with the different muscles and with the frequency of their activity. Generally, for example, the extensors react more quickly than the flexors. Furthermore, relaxing, which is less natural, requires more time than contraction. The duration of the transmission of the nerve impulse is sufficient to account physiologically for the greater retardation of the contraction of a group of muscles farther away from the motor centres (muscles of the foot compared to muscles of the face, for example), or for the longer latent time of a reaction to a tactile excitation brought from the foot than from the face. In the same muscular group, the movement of retracting the hand is brought about more quickly to an electrical excitation than for a wholly artificial action in the opposite direction.

[3] Each individual requested to beat time as he wishes adopts a rhythm which is his own, and which varies little.

L

them are encountered only in so far as there has been special education (writing, musical execution, etc.).

The role of exercise in activity has often been studied, and the laws of progress through repetition have been made precise, thus duplicating the researches pursued from the point of view of mnemonic functions and learning. But in the phenomena of exercise during an activity regulated by an assignment, an imposed task, work, there is something besides the progress of training.

In fact, after a certain number of repetitions of a task which is always the same, the progress, at first rapid, dies out and comes to an end. The efficiency no longer increases with successive repetitions.

Moreover, in the course of one of these series of repetitions, of executions of the task, of one of these periods of work, it is found that the efficiency does not attain its maximum value immediately ; it increases at first and then undergoes oscillations, which are of a much longer period than those which we have noted in connection with the study of attention.

Kraepelin has attributed the variations of efficiency during work to a series of factors combining their opposed tendencies : incitement, warming-up, spurt, in particular end-spurt, habit, all positive factors, on one hand ; loss of incitement and fatigue, negative factors, on the other hand.

Thorndike has rightly criticized the whole theoretical interpretation of Kraepelin.   In fact a progressive growth in efficiency is found in the initial phase of work, in which the process of warming-up (*Anregung*) manifests itself at times somewhat irregularly ;   then a period of stable efficiency, always with long-period oscillations[1] of minimum amplitude (besides the short-period oscillations attributed to attention) ;   finally a period of fatigue in which the efficiency progressively decreases.

Whenever the subject knows that he is approaching the end of his task, there is generally a final renewal of efficiency, attributed by Kraepelin to a factor called " spurt "

[1] Foucault thinks that the rhythmic variation in the speed of work reveals a process of optimal regulation.

(*Antrieb*). It is known, however, that numerous dynamogenic factors can, during the stable period, and especially during the phase of fatigue, produce an increase of efficiency, at least momentarily. These include certain sensory stimuli, above all affective stimuli, such as exhortations, factors of rivalry, the interest of the spectators, suggestions, etc. The certainty that only a brief effort will be needed is also an effective stimulant, of the same order as the preceding. Certain depressive factors also play their part : weariness, discouragement, etc.

Fatigue is considered as a depressive factor, but the word conveys quite different meanings. There is the fatigue which means simply the progressive diminution of efficiency during prolonged work, a phenomenon of considerable practical importance.[1] Fatigue is also used to describe the particular impression which is experienced in prolonged work, and which differs very much in its nature depending upon the character of the work. This impression includes localized pains following restricted muscular effort ; general depression with more complex work ; impressions of breathlessness, palpitation, etc., after very violent effort, like a race ; and disgust, nausea, headaches, visual troubles, profound ennui following purely intellectual work. Finally under the term fatigue are included general modifications of the organism following intense and prolonged work, varying with the nature of the work. Certain of these modifications are the source of very strongly felt impressions. These latter may arise from diffusion of effort, increased needs for energy, toxic agents carried around by the blood, etc.

[1] Consequently there is need to avoid the diminution of efficiency brought about by fatigue in order to maintain the output in industrial work and also in the field of scholarship. Researches have been started in both of these directions, from the point of view of the duration of work, the role of periods of rest, their frequency, length, etc. It is necessary in these researches to take account at the same time of the gain through interest and the loss by fatigue in order to discover the optimal distributions. Thus in the work of addition, it is unfavourable, with durations as short as 15 minutes, to have phases of work and rest excessively sub-divided ; whereas after 30 minutes' work, 5 minutes' rest is useful and still more, 15 minutes, after an hour (Amberg). Under other circumstances, after 30 minutes of intense work, one hour of rest is necessary (Rivers and Kraepelin).

In fact, in the course of continued work,[1] efficiency cannot be equally maintained ; it declines after a certain time even with constant effort. This is probably due in part to toxic effects caused by the waste products of metabolism produced in the course of muscular or nerve action, on the one hand, and, on the other, to the excessive consumption of reserves of energy, which are not replaced quickly enough, and which tend to become exhausted. These two categories of factors act unequally, depending upon the amount and the speed of the work.

An increase of effort, under the influence of external or purely mental dynamogenic stimulations, may counterbalance in a certain measure the loss by fatigue. This will be more difficult, at greater cost, and for a shorter time, as the fatigue becomes greater. Moreover, after the same length of time, the efficiency finally falls still lower, revealing a greater fatigue, caused by intoxication or exhaustion.

In turn there is often a letting-up in effort when the efficiency tends to diminish, which still further accelerates this diminution. The decrease in effort is demanded by the first characteristic impressions of the process of fatigue.[2]

When attempting to maintain a continuous effort of maximal compression of the hand on the bulb of the dynamograph, it is definitely found that the lowering of efficiency, which is here immediate, may be seen to follow a concave curve whenever the diminution of effort anticipates the loss of muscular efficiency (possibly with the continuation of a weak habit of control for a long time),

---

[1] In case of periodic work, like that of the heart, if the rhythm is slow enough, the work may be continued almost indefinitely without fatigue, for example, work on the ergograph with a light enough weight and sufficient interval between the contractions. The more rapid the rhythm, the earlier is the fatigue and the less the total output. Speed is also costly in human work, moreover, it is more costly as it more nearly approaches its limit.

[2] It is sometimes supposed that this initial lowering of efficiency results normally from an inhibiting reflex action, even when no impression of fatigue is perceived. Fatigue certainly should include this inhibition, which is intended to prevent exhaustion or toxic action (which others consider to be the fatigue).

or it may follow a convex form whenever the loss of efficiency is relatively compensated by a continued increase in effort up to the point of sudden and total surrender (see Fig. 9). Intermediate forms are observed between these types, but a progressive lowering of efficiency with the maintenance of constant effort is rare.

The cessation of work is followed by recuperation and a return to the initial state. This means the elimination of toxic products and the re-establishment of the energy reserves, a return to physiological equilibrium by the dying out of vascular and cardiac perturbations, etc. Efficiency is re-established at its original level, even if not at a higher level, from the advance made by practice.

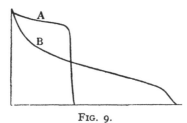

FIG. 9.

Two opposite types of dynamographic curves. In A is shown the " convex " type, in B the " concave " type.

When work is undertaken again before recuperation is complete, fatigue comes more quickly and is overcome with more difficulty.

By the continuation of successive periods of work without complete recuperation, physiological modifications are produced which disturb the normal equilibrium and constitute the state of overwork.

The state of overwork may be brought about by the mere prolongation of such sensori-motor activity as is characteristic of being awake, so that the repose of natural sleep is not allowed to occur with adequate regularity and duration.[1] This overwork is the most frequent among

[1] After prolonged insomnia a toxic substance develops which selectively attacks the cells of the cerebral cortex and prevents their functioning (the hypnotoxin of Piéron and Legendre).

children of school age when intellectual activity is added to physical activity.[1]

[1] There is really no balancing of these two forms of activity, in spite of what is often claimed. Fatigue due to one of these forms of work is increased by activity of the other form. Effort in physical activity, including as it does the regulation of the control of the muscles, always represents a cerebral activity, identical in nature with that which results from intellectual work.

Chapter III

THE HIERARCHY OF ACTS

VOLUNTARY ACTIVITY AND SOCIAL BEHAVIOUR

THE different activities may be classified according to their varying complexity and difficulty, which are in evidence whenever mental force is reduced, in the states known as neurasthenic and psychasthenic. Pierre Janet has traced, in a very interesting way, an entire hierarchy of behaviour according to the sort of damage to the activities thus affected.

The easiest acts are those which do not have to take account of the resistances of the environment, the physical environment and especially the social milieu (the social surroundings of most students make adaptation exceedingly difficult). One such type of activity is that of reverie, in which the activity is carried out exclusively in the sphere of the imagination.

But reverie may be carried on at very different levels ; it may be reduced to approach modes of purely automatic association[1] reaching the extremely loose association of the dream, in which there is no stable direction, or, on the contrary, it may rise towards creative thought, capable of bringing forth fruitful inventions.

Purely rational regulative action may encounter obstacles and resistances in the automatic tendencies, the desires, the affective impressions. Scientific thought, aiming to attain objective truth by the proven procedures of logic, which social education provides, is at a particularly high level. If there is slackness of thought, affective

---

[1] In which case associations of a lower order predominate, as in the logorrhoea of maniacs, a succession of assonances, verbal resemblances, or habitual chance associations.

logic of an opposite sort predominates. This permits immediate mental satisfaction with the announcement of ready-made opinions unrestrained by logical criticism, as in the modes of thought of primitive minds.

In the lower levels of mental activity " suggestion " acts most easily. It utilizes tendencies that are already prepared, thoughts all made, economizes effort and is in general accord with slack behaviour.

There are not only variable levels of efficiency (levels of attention) for a given activity, but the forms of activity tend to be transformed when the general level of efficiency is lowered. Certain activities, normally inhibited, are then liberated and carried as far as the lowering of the level of efficiency permits.[1] As certain automatic acts reveal the death agony, when the higher control fails, so mere depression through fatigue, through emotional shock, through intoxication, through nervousness, permits tics to appear which are otherwise repressed.

The automatisms of habit, activities often repeated, which gain exercise easily from the fact of this repetition (by virtue of the general law of mnemonic acquisition), direct all motor energy toward their pathways of less resistance.

Automatic activity and voluntary activity are thus generally opposed.

In this sense intentional activity is regarded as voluntary. Besides the reflex responses directly connected to stimuli, automatic activities which are blind and have power to develop, there exist acts which are characteristic of the psychological level of activity. These forms of conduct result from the play of the mass of mental functions, and express the personality, the unity of the individual.

Among these forms of activity, there are derivatives which imply the representation of an end, pre-vision—at

[1] According to Pierre Janet, efficiency is a function of the harmonious combination of what is called psychical force and tension. The automatisms of the maniac reveal an excess of energy when the tension is low. It requires at the same time high tension and a large amount of energy in order to sustain the highest levels of efficiency.

least approached—of consequences. Compared with associations of the low level, voluntary mental activity has the appearance of being regulated by a real command.

What, we may ask, is the nature of intentional activities in their motor aspect? They are essentially complex activities, perceptive adaptations. As we have already indicated, a person does not voluntarily contract an isolated muscle of the arm or hand, he gives a punch or he takes an object.

Moreover, certain acts which are useless for man are now beyond his powers, like the movement of the outer ear; movements of the head alone assure him of auditory orientation, although in many mammals it is still the movement of the external ear which occurs, the head remaining relatively still.

But just as special perceptive education permits the knowledge of forms or of separate colours and not only of objects, so motor education permits acrobats to accomplish isolated movements with different groups of muscles.[1] Certain people readily acquire the ability to move their ears at will, through systematic training which is founded on groping trials among which the successful ones are selected.

Voluntary activity is the connection of a mental elaboration with movements, the translation of thought into acts. It is not the direct incitations conveyed to the muscles after a representation of their action, but is the liberation of motor mechanisms already prepared by heredity or by habit. In the case of habits these mechanisms are acquired after groping activities, the importance and continuance of which we see during childhood. This voluntary motor activity may be compared to the action of a pianola on which the perforated rolls are changed, and which is regulated, and has its mechanism accelerated or retarded and its action released or stopped, by the use of

[1] A certain professional " phenomenon," by displacing his deltoid muscle and subluxation of the head of the humerus, can elongate his arm 4 or 5 cm., show a displaced epigastric arch, imitate the abdomen of a pregnant woman by producing an infra-umbilical prominence, etc. He commenced his apprenticeship at the age of eleven.

the pedals. There is found in commerce, that is to say in the normal framework of habitual mechanisms, only a complication of parts. If it is desired to play a scale, to sound separate notes, these particular perforated bands can only be prepared by a long and difficult process. So it is with the acrobats we spoke of above, and when they prepare their nerve pathways.

The force and speed of movements still depend upon voluntary regulation, but in their medium amounts only. Thus if, during an act of lifting, the resistance is suddenly varied, there is an increase in the force of contraction which is purely reflex. Its very short latent time indicates that it is regulated by a medullary reaction.

Effort, says Morgan, is the response to a checking stimulus ; in this sense there is even reflex effort, infra-psychic.

When a person proceeds at a certain speed to carry out a quite simple act, to trace a line or to write a letter, it is found that the speed increases regularly during the first part of the act, remains constant for about two-thirds, then decreases to the end.[1] This variation is not voluntary ; it is not even recognized.

There is a regulation of movement which is based entirely on the activity itself. In tabes, locomotion is not co-ordinated (locomotor ataxy), because the pathways of transmission for centripetal impulses, which carry kinæsthetic impressions, are interrupted. Mental control through vision may take their place to a certain extent, but the control of kinæsthetic origin is reflex and infra-psychic. Whenever the kinæsthetic perceptions are lost, in cerebral anæsthesia through limited lesions of the cortex (around the Post-Rolandic convolution), locomotor inco-ordination is not found, the reflex co-ordination remains assured through the lower levels.

[1] This is what Binet and Courtier, among other writers, have clearly established by the use of Edison's ingenious electric pen. This S-shaped curve of the speed of movements has been interpreted by Brailsford Robertson as characteristic of a type of physico-chemical reaction which corresponds to voluntary activity. But any motor which starts and stops has also an S-shaped curve representative of speeds.

Voluntary activity releases or stops, re-enforces or moderates an act as a whole ; it accelerates or retards the general pace of movements.   It has no value except as a means of regulation, within certain limits of force and speed.[1]

All the above concerns voluntary activity conceived as conduct, as intentional activity.   But in the hierarchy of acts, the term voluntary is often reserved for those responses which correspond to the highest steps, to the most difficult acts.

In the elaboration preceding a decision, a conflict of tendencies may be presented.   If there are certain tendencies towards immediate satisfactions in opposition to tendencies which present different satisfactions (success in an examination involving tedious work in place of taking a pleasant walk, for example), the conduct is regarded as corresponding better to a " voluntary " act, since it will result in a more marked predominance of more intellectual tendencies.[2]

Whenever the conflict brings about a contest between individual, egoistic tendencies and social tendencies (causing conveniences, juridical rules, moral traditions, etc., to intervene) that conduct is considered most volun-

---

[1] The slowness, as well as the speed of a movement, is limited, with certain differences depending upon the nature of the movements.   For the most rapid displacements of the arms which it is possible to execute (the maximum speed depending upon the direction of the displacement), about 0·3 second is required for 10 cm. displacement.   The greater the extent of the movement the greater its rapidity may be.   A displacement of 10 cm. does not require twice the time necessary for a displacement of 1 cm.

The maximum speed of successive movements, as to the number per second, is about 5 for the arm (shoulder), 6 for the jaw, 7 for flexing the foot, 11 for the hand (wrist), tapping with a pencil or with the finger on a telegraph key.   The typewriting record corresponds to 8 or 9 taps per second, but this is a complex task.   In trills on the piano, 15 or 16 notes are the extreme limit with two fingers, making a maximum of 8 taps for one finger.

[2] The idea of volition has also a moral significance, and is closely connected, from this point of view, with the idea of responsibility.   But psychology is not concerned with this aspect of the idea.   The psychologist makes no distinction between Mucius Scaevola putting his hand in the flame in order to prove his fearlessness, and a highway robber, in order not to betray himself, bandaging up a wound, while concealing the terrible pain caused by being shot in his stomach.

tary which yields to the most sublimated tendencies, that is to say, the most social conduct.

This conception of the voluntary is not properly psychological ; it is founded on the idea of value and corresponds to a hierarchical classification of individual acts and individuals themselves. We shall return later to this idea of volition, approaching it from the idea of intelligence, both of which ideas have an exclusively practical interest.

PART SIX

MENTAL STAGES AND TYPES

CHAPTER I

MENTAL EVOLUTION AND LEVELS OF DEVELOPMENT

AT birth the infant lives by means of its hereditary equipment of reflexes and elementary instincts. From the first minutes of life, moreover, according to the many observations by Margaret Gray Blanton, there may be observed among certain new-born infants, tears, cries, yawns, starting at a noise, rotation of the head, defending the respiration when the infant is placed on its face, fixation of a light, and even a movement of following the hand with the eye (generally later). Naturally there is an immediate sucking activity permitting the infant placed at the breast to nourish itself, precocious movements of feeling for the breast, a clasping reflex (the fist closes and holds tight at any excitation of the palm), etc.

At this time a large number of nerve paths are not yet functioning. Their fibres have not yet acquired their myelin sheaths. The higher centres of the cortex as yet play no part. But there is quite marked inequality in nerve development among the new-born, even for those of full term.[1]

Affective expressions of satisfaction or pain are immedi-

[1] Mnemonic capacities of the nervous system manifest themselves very early, but the fixation of enduring memories is tardy. It is rare that any trace continues from the first two years, even with a child three years old. Memories are exceptional, among adolescents or adults, which go back to 16 or 20 months of age. I have heard a case cited of a memory from 10 months, but with no way of checking it.

ate, existing even among anencephalics reduced to a thalamic life. Apart from painful cutaneous sensibility, taste is the most precocious, at least in its affective manifestations.

The development of the child, in respect of physical growth and functional perfection, including progress through training, is accomplished with very great rapidity. The growth is most rapid at first, and then continues by a slower and slower rhythm until it becomes unnoticeable at the end of adolescence.

During babyhood, the perfecting of the nervous system first makes possible automatic activities like walking and preserving the equilibrium, also spatial reactions which become gradually more precise ; it assures the co-ordination of the movements and the more and more perfect unification of conduct (development of the attention, of voluntary motor activity, etc.), with the possibility of variable reactions ;[1] it permits also the appearance of spontaneous vocal play, which conditions these innate tendencies, and which contributes to the educative acquisition of language.

In fact, along with the spontaneous progress through exercise by play, elementary sensori-motor play, then more and more complex play, there is progress through the educative influence of the environment. This is relatively systematized and implies essentially the acquisition of the verbal instrument. Through the mechanism of conditioned reflexes, a certain number of the vocal sounds heard acquire value as signs, and become registered in memory. Among the spontaneous vocal sounds of the child he makes a selection of those which correspond to these signs. Language is thus born and develops, at a rate which accelerates at first and then retards. It follows the general form of the S-shaped curve characteristic of the processes of growth.

[1] Hunter shows that, from 13 to 16 months, an interval of 15 seconds between the perception of a dainty put in a box in the neighbourhood of two others and the natural attempt to open the box, is sufficient to cause errors in half the cases. Stability of attention and the maintenance of an attitude require greater maturity.

At a certain time, generally at the beginning of the second year, imitative play appears. This favours education in general and especially the acquisition of a vocabulary[1] and the formation of phrases (the word-phrase being the primitive verbal manifestation).[2] Although the verbal tool may be furnished the child by society, the utilization of this tool is not immediately socialized. Language is used at first for individual play. The monologues which are made up in the course of pseudo-conversation and approach a primitive form of thought, entirely escape the requirements of rigorous logic.

The mentality of a child, until about 7 years of age, is dominated by " egocentrism," as the excellent researches of Piaget well demonstrate.

The child, as the centre of the universe, takes himself as a type, as a model, and conceives everything in his own image, living as he does, acting with the same intentions as he does (whence arises animism, " magical " interpretations, etc.). At this time a motive appears as a necessary and sufficient cause.

Furthermore, the child's own creative activity encourages him to attribute origin by creation to all things. The questions of the child, " who made it and how ? " manifest his idea of the creation of animals, of children themselves, etc. At first everything possesses equivalent reality, the imaginative constructions of the dream as well as the waking perceptions. This should make the moralists cautious in regard to childish " lies."

---

[1] Thanks to methodical inventories of vocabularies, Mlle. Descoeudres furnishes the following indications of the increase in the number of words with age, a growth which is clearly represented by the S-curve : at 12 months 4 words ; at 15 months, 18 ; at 18 months, 48 ; at 21 months, 174 ; at 2 years 9 months, 639 ; at 3 years 10 months, 1,394 ; at 5 years, 1,954 ; at 7 years, 2,903. The dictionary includes nearly 40,000 words. The researches of a dozen authors fix at about ten words (between 3 and 24) the vocabulary at 1 year, at 1,600 (between 650 and 2,300) the vocabulary at 3 years. Apart from these facts the researches are much more uncertain. The usual vocabulary of a peasant does not exceed 3,000 words. When the average number of words understood at the end of development is estimated, the numbers vary between 8,000 and 20,000.

[2] For a child to say "hat" when learning to speak, means, for example : " Put on your hat and give me mine so that we can go for a walk."

The ideas of the child, confused and undifferentiated, partake, following the expression of Renan, of the primitive " syncretism " which characterizes perception. The attitudes and acts are moulded by objects, or better, by total situations which are not analysed, and which cannot be logically confronted.[1]

Starting at 7 years, in the second period of childhood, socialization really begins. Thanks to the verbal categories, the child accomplishes the work of analysis and synthesis, pulling apart and reconstructing objects and situations.[2] Egocentrism, or " autism," is restrained, only to reappear in pathological states like certain forms of dementia præcox. At the same time the play of the imagination is controlled and held back. But it is not until about 11 years, at the end of this second period, that formal thought becomes possible, that the utilization of true concepts begins, and that the knowledge of conventional time is really acquired.[3] Only at this age does the child become an incomplete adult, losing his initial peculiarities at the beginning of adolescence.[4]

Parallel to the intellectual evolution and to the progress of growth, there is an affective evolution. It manifests itself in the nature of the interests, which reveal the dominating tendencies.

[1] In this stage, when the logical instrument is not yet acquired by the child, there exists an " intelligent " capacity of reflection in regard to practical problems, which are solved through the benefit of individual experience. The child of three years is very superior to most animals, including the lower apes, so far as the methods which he uses to open a box the mechanism of which is hidden (Boutan).

[2] The drawings of the child are characterized by a realism which Luquet wrongly calls "logical." It consists in representing the object syncretically in all its complexity and not as visual analysis might reveal it. Visual " realism " is acquired at the same time as logical.

[3] Orientation in time, the acquisition of the first syncretic notions of space and time occurs at the age of 2 or 3 years. The notions of yesterday and to-morrow are but little understood before 5 years. Plurality is already observed at 2 years, groups of 4 objects are specifically recognized about 3 years, of 5 objects about 5 years. Arithmetic cannot be usefully taught in this precocious fashion, unless it becomes pure verbalism.

[4] An arrest of development at a stage below 3 years produces idiocy ; an arrest at a stage between 3 and 7 years inclusive produces corresponding levels of imbecility ; an arrest between 7 and 11 years a mental weakness, compatible, however, with social utilization.

The interests are sensori-motor until about 15 to 18 months, and they govern the play of elementary learning. The infant is sucker and beholder, then grabber, feeler, trotter. Finally come the so-called "subjective" interests, corresponding to infantile egocentrism, with the activity of the speaker, the constructor, the questioner. Little by little appear the more objective interests, and finally the social interests, the sex interests accompanying the efflorescence of puberty, when the affective exuberance overflows into æsthetic sentiments, poetic reveries, etc.

The freshness of the sentiments, the vivacity of the tendencies, corresponds to a marked predominance of the affective life in childhood and early youth, just as senile involution is above all characterized by affective enfeeblement.[1]

The rapidity of mental development is very unequal among children, as is the rapidity of physical growth, in height for example.[2] The differences are due on the one hand to an intrinsic factor related to the rapidity of evolution, and on the other to the whole capacity for development. Thus, for two children who attain the same height at the end of their growth, one may be more precocious than the other, his growth continuing a shorter time. However, usually in a homogeneous environment, a taller child than another will attain a greater height at the end of the period of growth. The mental level of development, which corresponds to the average of various functions, is like the physical level of development.[3]

Variability increases with age. According to measures

---

[1] The dying out of tendencies contributes to throw the aged back into the past; and moreover, since their mnemonic fixation is diminished, the old memories are most easily recalled.

[2] Mental development certainly corresponds to the growth of the brain, which, about 330 grams on the average at birth, nearly doubles in six months, reaches 990 grams at 2 years and 1,300 at 14 years, in progressing towards a final limit on the average of 1,375 grams.

[3] To Alfred Binet we are indebted for the first scales, empirically standardized, which permitted the mental ages of children to be measured and the degrees of mental retardation to be determined. The series of tests of Binet and Simon have played a considerable rôle in the evolution and spread psychometric methods.

M

carried out for a series of functions,[1] for classifying children according to their mental levels, it is established that the middle half, after eliminating the lowest quarter, and the highest quarter, is included at 7 years within an interval corresponding to about 16 months of age, at 14 years to an interval three times as great. Individual differences are, therefore, then more noticeable ; but the variability is often greater in appearance than in reality, since the absolute differences in age are then less.

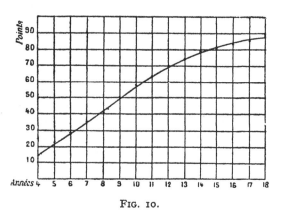

FIG. 10.

Curve of growth of mental level (evaluated in points) as a function of age, according to measurements made with the scale of Yerkes and Wood.

The progress of the average mental level (for sensori-motor, mnemonic, verbal, and logical functions, capacities of efficiency, etc.) is carried out according to the type of the S-curve ; but it reveals for certain functions, with certain tests, critical stages, in particular around 7 years and from 10 to 11 years, to which ages we have already called attention.

[1] The measure of development, while avoiding tests intended to call for acquisitions which result from a too special type of instruction (definite scholastic information, for example), is not able to eliminate entirely educational acquisition, since the normal development of a civilized child implies such education. It supposes then that the children compared have been submitted to the same educational influences. This postulate, which is approximately true for children of the same environment, limits the application of scales of measurement.

CHAPTER II

THE DIFFERENTIATION OF NATURAL TYPES

SEX AND RACE

WHEN the progress of mental development is followed, certain differences are noted in the general form of this progress, depending upon whether the children observed are in one environment or another, from one country or another, of this race or that, and also whether the boys and girls are examined separately. The differences in development which are noted among children submitted to similar or identical education are indications of mental differences betrayed among adults, from the point of view of the average level, and especially from the point of view of the mental type.

Actually, the same level of development may be encountered among very different individuals, at any age of childhood and at adult age. The superiority of one individual over another from the point of view of certain functions is set over against relative deficiencies.

One person has a very good memory and greater motor competence with somewhat unstable attention and mediocre intelligence, while another, attentive and intelligent, has deficiencies of memory and is notably clumsy.

The analytical determination of the mental type permits the measurement of such differences, which characterize one group in comparison with another.

It is not sufficient to say that, in a general way, girls are more precocious than boys. Their advantage is especially noticeable beginning at 7 years and continuing until 14 or 15 years, but since the slowing up of their development comes earlier, it is such that the advantage diminishes and disappears, to give place to a slight inferiority of the average level at the approach of adult age.

In fact, this difference in rate of mental development, just as in physical development, is superimposed on the more marked differences in the average mental type. The feminine sex shows a richer imagination, a much greater emotivity, with some affective instability, more accentuated suggestibility, more docility, regularity in attentive effort, capacity for automatization. Dexterity and the aptitude for acquiring languages also correspond to feminine superiorities.[1]

On the other hand, the masculine type possesses a more coherent logic, a more marked power of invention and of intellectual creativeness, a greater capacity for abstraction, more courage, initiative, moderation and balance. Variability is greater among homogeneous groups of men than of women.

These differences characterize the average masculine and feminine types in the same way that man is said to be taller than woman as regards height. But the superposition of the frequency curves is such that it is also true that a large number of men are shorter than the average of the women and a large number of women taller than the average of the men. Similarly many men will be found more emotional, more suggestible and more imaginative than the average woman, and many women more logical, more inventive and more courageous than the average man. The average differences between the sexes imply only that, in submitting a group composed of an equal number of men and women to the same selection tests, there will be found proportionally more men than women

---

[1] Heymans, in the course of statistical researches through inquiries based on questionnaires, found that it is in emotivity and activity that the feminine mentality essentially differs from the masculine. The traits of character derived from these, which are more frequent in the female are : inconstancy of mood, anxiety, faint-heartedness, persistence of sadness, brevity of anger, need for change, propensity to laugh, shortcomings in logic, repugnance to abstraction, intuitive thought, aptitude for languages, impulsiveness, fanaticism, dexterity, vanity, a dominating spirit, a penchant for exaggeration, excess of cruelty and of pity, interest in religion, mental instability, sincerity, a tendency to economy, patience during illness.

or more women than men, depending upon the requirements of the selection, who will be classed in the first half or the first quarter of the group.

Education, environment, tradition and custom play an important role in the genesis of these average differences between men and women, varying in regard to the particular characteristics which are favoured or restrained.[1] However, with the same education, there remain, in the nature of the intelligence, and above all in the affectivity and character, certain differences which depend upon physiological influences of sexual origin. The effects of castration or of genital grafts, the consequences of certain glandular disturbances, have shown the place of internal secretions connected with the genital functions in the genesis of the pride and aggressiveness of the male, as well as in the docility and coquetry of the female.

The action of the sex instinct corresponds to the different behaviour of the two sexes. During gestation and after the birth of a child, the maternal instinct in woman, which also has a physiological origin, is manifested even without the influence of tendencies of social origin which favour the family and are instilled through education.

When, in turn, not individuals of the two sexes in the same environment are compared, but individuals belonging to different environments, it is more difficult to determine what is due to educational differences and what to fundamental special traits.

What is called national character is, for the most part, a question of educational tradition, and any individual placed in the same environment will receive the national imprint. As regards the origin of these educational traditions, however, it is necessary to recognize more fundamental differences of social types.

---

[1] Heymans has devoted attention to the role of sexual selection in certain feminine traits. In particular there seems to be a temporary effect of masculine taste on the behaviour of young girls, who, at one time, will exaggerate their lack of courage and capriciousness in order to be more feminine, and, at another, will be more masculine in order to be companions of men.

Among the white, yellow and black races there are, in the type of intelligence and in the character, differences which are observable even when the education has been identical. The black race in particular is more precocious, but its period of development is less prolonged, so that the average level of the adult is lower. In the yellow race there does not appear to be a characteristic difference in this respect from the whites. Furthermore, the black race is more unstable, more concrete in its thinking ; the yellow race has an affective life that is more balanced, more matter of fact.[1]

Among whites the racial differences are quite difficult to state precisely because of the intermixing which has singularly blended Germans, Celts, Latins and even Slavs. Nevertheless, among the racial characteristics within the national group, which is always relatively heterogeneous, there is always discovered relatively greater precocity of development, especially in the southern races, showing itself in the average mental level of adults, in the more imaginative or more abstract type of intelligence, in the more gay and expansive or more sad and reserved character. The Latin type, the Semitic type, and the Slav type, in particular, are well distinguished.

But the fundamental differences of hereditary types are often insignificant compared with the differences due to the type of civilization and level of culture.

The Asiatic civilization turned towards the traditional culture of the past, which expressed itself concretely in

[1] It was at first sought to discover differences among the races in their elementary processes, especially in their sensations. Only insignificant differences were found. But the perceptive education necessary to the conditions of life in primitive surroundings (the necessity of procuring food by hunting and fishing, of defence against wild beasts and enemies, etc.) produces a notable superiority, compared with that in the civilized environment, in the capacity to interpret visual, auditory and olfactory impressions, to orient themselves, etc. The defects of language, the symbolic instrument, which economizes memories among civilized people, necessitate a greater appeal among primitive peoples to mnemonic registration and a better utilization of concrete memories. Habits also cause different likes and dislikes, that is to say, quite other affective influences from certain impressions of taste and odour. The absence of interest in analytic differentiation carries with it among primitive peoples a very feeble ability to differentiate colours and musical tones.

the worship of ancestors. This impressed on the Chinese mentality a very special character favourable to æsthetic creation, but not capable of being brought within our logic and our science, the abstract concepts of which find no place at all in the infinitely blended expressions of their language.

The effect on the individual of the structure of collective traditions, closely connected with the verbal instrument in which they are expressed, gives to primitive peoples a mentality exclusively based on magical beliefs and impervious to experience. It persists in our modern civilizations only a very rudimentary form and in country environments deprived of instruction.

CHAPTER III

THE HIERARCHIC ARRANGEMENT OF
INDIVIDUALS AND JUDGMENTS OF VALUE

WILL—INTELLIGENCE

WHEN the progress of mental development is followed, it is considered as a whole. By appropriate tests directed at different functions, an average level is experimentally established, which increases with age to a relatively high limit, depending upon the individuals concerned.

But superiority of this mental level does not play a very great practical role in our social organization which is founded on a division of work. We can quite well determine hierarchies among individuals ; we evaluate, we compare, we classify, but always from a quite special point of view.[1] For example, when considering feminine charm in a beauty competition, or physical vigour in athletic contests, however varied, we evaluate skill, strength of will (energy, moral force, etc.), and intelligence. We seek to establish selections founded on the relative value of individuals from one of these points of view.

Rational, theoretical points of view, corresponding to a scientific attitude, are not here involved, but only practical points of view corresponding to the needs of social utilization.

The word " will " does not apply to an individualized mental function, but conceals a judgment of value expressed about conduct in all its complexity, a moral judgment.

[1] A person who is on the whole mediocre may sometimes be classed first according to points, in a contest based on many heterogeneous tests, while his specialized excellencies, if handicapped by the fact of complementary inferiorities, will leave him at least mediocre. This is too often forgotten in our scholastic estimates.

To have a strong will implies not only a high level of individualization of behaviour and a superior amount of mental energy, but a predominance of tendencies which are considered superior ; that is to say, of tendencies developed by society in the direction of its ideal, altruistic tendencies, socialized, sublimated, over tendencies considered inferior, appropriate tendencies for an individual, egoistic tendencies, biological, profoundly anchored in the organism.

The person who is capable of sustained effort in the satisfaction of his wants, in obeying his desires and his passions, in obtaining personal satisfactions, cannot be compared with one who shows the ability to repress his appetite for life, his instinct for self-preservation in danger, to cover up his sufferings and to sacrifice himself with a smile.

Will in this last case does not represent a mental function, but expresses a judgment of value concerning certain extremely complex conduct.

Paradoxical as it may seem at first, the same thing is true for intelligence,[1] which is the basis of hierarchies frequently established in our society.

In psychology superiority of intelligence[2] is often described as superiority of mental level, either among adults or among children of a given age. In the latter case, moreover, the greatest precocity is not always a sure precursor of definite superiority. However, there is a confusion here which results from our habit of speaking of intelligence when building up a mental hierarchy. It is necessary at least to make certain corrections,[3] in order to recall that intelligence as thus used is not what is ordinarily thought of as intelligence, that the same " value " is not under consideration.

[1] We leave out of consideration the use, borrowed from faculty psychology, of the words *will* and *intelligence* in psychological classification to refer to large groups of processes.

[2] The American psychologists tend also to describe as a " genius " a child who has, at a given mental age, a certain advance in mental age, in its level of development, above the average level.

[3] Claparède distinguishes this sort of intelligence under the name " global," in opposition to what he calls " integral " intelligence.

In current judgment, anyone is considered intelligent who comprehends quickly and well, or who manifests a cautious critical mind, or again, who shows creative capacities and produces fruitful inventions or distinguished work.

Capacities of comprehension, of criticism, of invention, in the course of thought, as we have indicated, are necessary to solve problems. In reality it is the general capacity to solve difficulties, to attack new situations with success, to disentangle matters under unusual circumstances,[1] which is appreciated under the name intelligence.

Thus, in our hierarchy of animal species, as we have already noted, we oppose intelligence to instinct, as a plastic capacity for adaptation to new circumstances to the routine automatism of perfect execution under identical conditions, which fails under the slightest change.

When it is desired to compare intelligences, the tests to which individuals are submitted always consist of problems proposed to them.[2]

But the solution of problems does not depend upon a separable function of "intelligence," which can be psychologically defined; it is the organization of a complex activity in which the whole mental life may be brought to bear. The superiority of an individual depends not solely upon the greater development of certain mental functions, but upon the harmonious action of all the functions and a well-directed co-ordination of mental effort. This implies the essential intervention also of the affective life and interests.[3]

Though we always employ the same word, intelligence,

[1] Auguste Comte early said that intelligence is "the aptitude for modifying conduct so as to conform to the circumstances of each case."

[2] In classification, the speed of solution is generally regarded as of first importance. Although speed is of great practical importance in a large number of cases, in others it is negligible, and it is the idea of power, of profundity, based upon the degree of maximum difficulty which can be overcome without limit of time, which alone should be considered.

[3] Thus, in the analytic definitions of the process of intelligence, besides the steps of comprehension (stating the problem), of invention (imagining a solution), and of criticism (verifying the solution), about which most psychologists are agreed (Binet, Claparède, etc.), the notion of direction is frequently introduced (Binet), or of interest (Heymans), or of curiosity (Woodworth). These indicate the indispensable role of actors of affective regulation.

for the aptitude to solve problems, it is still necessary to understand that under this term the mental action may be quite different, depending upon the nature of the problems to be solved, just as the term athletic ability, depending upon the nature of the contest, includes jumping, throwing the discus, track events, field events, etc. There are really many forms of intelligence covering very different mental processes.[1]

The problems that we may have to solve are very different in nature. They concern our direct contacts with the things we have to manage, with the physical environment in which we live, or our relations with men and with the social environment, or again, our manipulation of the concepts which we have acquired and which we wish to assure ourselves are logically treated, or finally our contacts with the mass of images which we have stored up and which we can reconstruct.

The mechanician who must assemble the pieces of a machine in a desired manner, the guide who must orient himself in little known regions, the executive who must solve all the difficulties which pertain to the management of a heterogeneous personnel, the statesman who would convince an assembly, the mathematician who pursues a symbolic deduction, the physicist who seeks the cause of a phenomenon, the philosopher who speculates on abstract conceptions, the architect who constructs a plan conforming to certain ends and meeting certain conditions, the musician who composes a symphony or the sculptor who produces a statue—each has to prove his intelligence, but it is a specialized intelligence and by no means interchangeable. The classification of all intelligent men will be very different according to the nature of the problems which may be chosen for the tests to which they are submitted.[2]

[1] In each form of intelligence, there are besides, as we shall note later, predominant types, those who comprehend better, are more inventive, or more critical.

[2] Among these forms of intelligence—mechanical, artistic, etc.—are those which are concrete, perceptive, imaginative; there are others which are essentially verbal, others also symbolic (mathematical) but using different symbols. In aphasia, the verbal and symbolic forms of intelligence are attacked.

Again, in order to make appropriate selections, the point of view of intelligence, which is of capital importance, since superiority in innovation means so much to our forms of society, ought to be specialized in the proper direction. There is too great a tendency, scholastic in origin, to consider only the logical and verbal form of intelligence.[1]

Finally, it is useful to carry through an analysis of intelligence, showing the relatively marked prominence of functions of comprehension, of invention, of criticism, of management, sometimes becoming stubbornness (out of which arises genius, " long patience "), the roles of speed and of profundity in the solution of problems, the more intuitive type of thought or the more analytic, the more affective, or the more logical, etc.

In order to provide for the division of work in society, it is necessary to define the common hierarchies and to appeal to analytic classifications which permit a suitable use of the aptitudes of each person.

---

[1] Sometimes in scholastic surroundings, intelligence is also confused with superior success in processes of acquisition or docility, and memory plays an essential role. Memory does not guarantee the capacity to solve problems of a new type when the use of learned formulæ is no longer sufficient. Thanks to these formulæ, in fact, to routine mechanisms, a person learns to solve problems of the current type without the need of intelligence. One of the purposes of education consists in thus making up for a deficiency of intelligence by memory ; but the essential aim is the opposite. It consists in making up for a deficiency of memory by intelligence, thus following the general trend of intellectual life in our European civilizations.

Chapter IV

THE ANALYTIC CLASSIFICATION OF INDIVIDUALS

TYPE—CHARACTER—MENTAL PROFILE

It is a fact of common observation that, under the same conditions, individuals who have received the same education nevertheless behave in quite different ways, each thinking and acting in his own manner.

This shows that even in a homogeneous group of men or of women, both from the ethnic or national standpoint, and from the point of view of their surroundings (urban or country) and of their social level, there exist notable differences, corresponding to types of individuals which are relatively well characterized.

The determination and the classification of these types is the purpose of researches which are grouped under the title differential psychology (W. Stern) or individual psychology (A. Binet). This heading is sometimes subdivided into ethology,[1] or the study of characters, and noology (Mentré), or the study of intelligences. These two branches cannot, however, be so arbitrarily separated, since they are unified in the personal regulation of behaviour in all its forms.

We have to do here, in reality, with a branch of descriptive anthropology which defines human groups under their morphological aspects as well as under their functional aspects, physiological and psychological. Within the social groups it sets up a classification of varieties forming sub-groups. These varieties, moreover,

---

[1] J. S. Mill employed this term " ethology," conceiving it especially as the science of the laws for the formation of character, for pedagogical use.

are more numerous and complex when the older strains are themselves more mixed, as is the case in most European countries and in American nations built up through immigration.

In our populations, an attempt has been made to distinguish human types whose physical characteristics should have functional and mental correlates : often on the hypothesis that the theoretical conception is that psycho-physiological characters were dependent on the morphological traits.

This theory is clearly related to the ancient doctrine of temperaments, which divided individuals into the sanguine, the nervous, the bilious and lymphatic (or phlegmatic).[1] It is often sought to fit celebrated personages into these groups, and to deduce the essential facts of their histories from appropriate laws of their temperaments. It is also common to believe that the intelligence can be judged according to features of the face and character estimated from the physiognomy, but there is little encouragement from the large percentage of errors found in the attempts at experimental verification.

There may actually be some correlations between the varieties of morphological constitution, between inequalities in the functional development of certain organs on the one hand and certain traits of character on the other. But when we enquire about the nature of these correlations, we are still almost always ignorant. There may be relations of cause and effect, as when it is known, for example, that bad functioning of the liver does not predispose to good humour and optimism ; or of simple coincidence, which may be repeated, as happens with two ethnic characters often transmitted together when a definite hereditary predominance is manifested in a type of mixed origin ; or, finally, a real but indirect relationship, when two different effects are manifested from the

[1] Classifications have recently been proposed which are more properly morphological. They refer to respiratory, digestive, muscular and cerebral types, always including general characterizations of these types from all points of view. According to Naccarati, emotional individuals would be those in whom the trunk is more developed than the limbs.

same cause, as when " virility " of character accompanies, for example, a considerable development of the hairy system, through the action of certain internal secretions, and both likewise occur among very young girls following an hypertrophy of the adrenal glands.

As far as that which concerns the character, the tendencies, the affective elements of conduct, we are sure, from numerous examples, that the main role is played by organic factors connected especially with the vegetative nervous system[1] and the endocrine balance. But we are not really ready to define character in organic terms. The young analytic science of man is not yet sufficiently developed.[2]

Many are content to describe and to classify. Characters are distinguished by one author as apathetic, sensitive, emotive, and passionate, with many variations (Malapert), besides amorphous or unstable types, and mixed types[3]

Another (Mentré) describes the practical intellectual type (the technician or administrator), the contemplative (intuitive, lyric—orator, poet, musician—or plastic), the abstract meditative (jurist or analyst) and the imaginative (geometrician or naturalist).

Frequently literary intelligence is distinguished from scientific, concrete from verbal, critical from creative (the flowering of which is genius), and the latter from merely comprehensive intelligence ; rapid intelligence is

[1] A quite general antagonism in functional regulation, between the sympathetic system and the para-sympathetic, has led to the distinction of two different types which are revealed especially by the oculo-cardiac reflex (slowing of the heart through releasing the inhibiting action of the vagus nerve when the eye is compressed), the " sympatheticotonics " and the " vagotonics." The predisposition to anxiety occurs in connection with vagotonic action, or at least in connection with a certain lack of balance which is expressed by alternate predominance, that of the vagus manifesting itself at the moment of crises of anguish.

[2] An American author has not hesitated to reproduce even to-day, under endocrine types, all the exaggerations of the theory of temperaments. He has described the famous men by a glandular formula, regarding them as hyperthyroid, hyposuprarenal, pituitary personalities, etc. (Berman). Napoleon is thus classified from this viewpoint as a pituitocentric.

[3] Ribot classified characters as sensitive, active, and apathetic, with the groups sensitive-active, apathetic-active, apathetic-sensitive, and mixed. Perez enumerates the quick, the quick ardent, the ardent, the slow, the slow ardent and the balanced.

distinguished from slow, reflective from inspirational,[1] etc.

The dreamer is set over against the man of action, and it is noted that the exaggeration of these types is shown in the domain of pathology (Kretschmer). The first, called "introverted," becomes a "schizoid," while the other, the "extraverted," or the "syntone," is attacked by obsessions or paranoia. In this field, the psychology of constitutions and types joins pathology.

Furthermore, in all functional researches, the distinction of different types is needed. From the point of view of attention, the capacity to direct and unify conduct, types are differentiated as of broad or narrow capacity, as quick or slow, sensory or motor, visual, auditory, etc., in accordance with the conditions of superiority required for efficiency (McComas).

In effort, as shown on the dynamograph, different types are very clearly observed, corresponding to certain forms of character, as we have already indicated in connection with activity (Part V, Chap. II).

In imagination and memory the predominance of different senses may be distinguished (visual, auditory, kinæsthetic).

But it must be recognized that these various individual characteristics cannot be grouped in well-defined types having an actual existence as the species were supposed to have in the old zoology with its impassable compartments.[2]

There are certain relatively frequent combinations of different characteristics, and we shall be better informed when we know what are the real relations, through direct kinship or collateral, what are the causes of certain

---

[1] This distinction is often made in the comparison of the classicists and the romanticists. Following Pascal, Poincaré and Duhem agree as to a three-fold division of learned men : the analysts (the rigorous minds of Pascal) the geometricians (broad-minded according to Duhem), and finally the idealists (minds with fine appreciation according to Pascal).

[2] In constructing types of character with a claim to absolute value, the division into faculties, with its juxtaposed entities in the mind, has naturally been utilized. Individuals have then been distinguished according to the predominance of intellect, feeling or will.

habitual coincidences, and what are the principal independent traits to consider.

Meanwhile, we can only reason statistically and consider
empirically the chances of association of two characteristics, according to the frequency of their occurrence.

This requires many systematic investigations, which are
not yet available, but will multiply in view of practical
needs.

Indeed the growing movement for a rational utilization
of individuals in accordance with a well-conducted
professional orientation, will make it necessary to provide

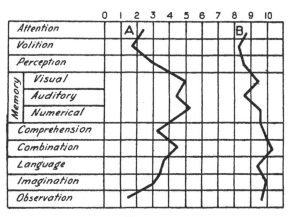

FIG. 11.

Two mean psychological "profiles" determined by Rossolimo. On the
one hand a group of children who are mentally retarded is shown by
curve A, on the other a group of well-endowed children by curve B.

for each individual a chart of his organic activity, both
physiological and psychological.   This will offer study
material of the first importance for individual psychology.

In particular the use of the mental profile (see Fig. 11),
an ingenious idea which occurred to Rossolimo, gives a
graphic representation of an individual, which facilitates
the comparison, grouping and classification of types.   A
better idea of the possibilities of success in life can thus be
gained through the definition of aptitudes.   At first the
descriptions will be empirical, but they will undoubtedly

N

be rationalized little by little with the growth of knowledge.[1]

The characteristics of creative genius—which is bound to imply a large amount of dreaming favourable to original inspiration[2]—will undoubtedly betray themselves among adolescents in a manner sufficiently precocious for the birth of fruitful inventions to be aided.[3]

Already the differentiation of various retarded types of the mentally weak (the mentally deficient)—a more easy task—permits the maximum utilization of the limited aptitudes of these sub-normals.[4] Moreover, they are sometimes more able than more intelligent individuals to adapt themselves to certain automatic and monotonous tasks.

The practical applications of individual psychology have an importance which is gaining wider recognition every day. Psychometry, a special branch of anthropometry, plays the principal role in individual psychology, providing it with the numerical determinations which permit the construction of mental profiles.

[1] In the characterization of types, even from the point of view of intellectual behaviour, the whole personality must be considered ; the character, the tendencies and the affective elements also intervene to determine the form of intelligence. The interests combine with the mental aptitudes, and tastes enter into the conduct of thought.

[2] An excess of voluntary action in thought, of attentive unification, is opposed to truly original and new associative groupings and to inspiration, which, by contact with streams of ideas or images, permits invention, real creation.

[3] It is not through individual biographies of genius that there will be the best chance of discovering the key to genius, unless such monographs become numerous enough to permit the general relations to be discovered by statistical methods. Without this it is a risk to give importance to characteristic insignificant traits which are met by chance. Centenarians thus attribute their remarkable longevity to their own particular *régime* ; some are abstainers, others smoke and drink their daily glass of spirits.

[4] Exact knowledge of the mental functions of those who have sensory abnormalities, the blind and the deaf-mutes, permits their education also to be directed in a more satisfactory manner, in order that their abilities may be better utilized in society.

BIBLIOGRAPHY

1.—TREATISES

DUMAS, GEORGES, with 24 collaborators, *Traité de Psychologie*, 2 vols., 8vo, Paris, 1923–4 ; 2nd ed., 6 vols., in Press.

EBBINGHAUS, H., *Grundzüge der Psychologie*, 3rd ed., Leipzig, 1913.

JAMES, W., *Principles of Psychology*, 2 vols., London and New York, 1890–2.

LADD and WOODWORTH, *Elements of Physiological Psychology*, 8vo, London, 1911.

LEHMANN, ALFRED, *Grundzüge der Psychophysiologie*, 8vo, Leipzig, 1912.

WUNDT, W., *Grundzüge der physiologischen Psychologie*, 5th ed., 3 vols., 8vo, Leipzig, 1915.

2.—OUTLINES AND MANUALS

EBBINGHAUS, H., *Abriss der Psychologie*, Leipzig, 1900.

HÖFFDING, H., *Outlines of Psychology*, trans. by M. E. Lowndes, London and New York, 1891.

JAMES, W., *Text Book of Psychology—Briefer Course*, 8vo, New York, 1908.

JUDD, C. H., *General Introduction to Psychology*, 8vo, New York, 1907.

McDOUGALL, W., *An Outline of Psychology*, 8vo, London, 1913.

PILLSBURY, W. S., *The Fundamentals of Psychology*, 8vo, New York, 1922.

TITCHENER, E. B., *A Text Book of Psychology*, 8vo, New York.

VAISSIÈRE, J. DE LA, *Éléments de Psychologie Expérimentale*, 8vo, Paris, 1912.

WARREN, H. C., *Human Psychology*, 8vo, Boston and New York, 1920.

WOODWORTH, R. S., *Psychology, A Study of Mental Life*, 8vo, London, 1922.

3.—WORKS ON TECHNICAL METHODS

GIESE, F., *Handbuch psychotechnischer Eignungsprüfungen*, 8vo, Halle, 1925.

LANGFELD, H. S. and ALLPORT, F. H., *An Elementary Laboratory Course in Psychology*, 8vo, Boston and New York, 1917.

MYERS, C. S., *Text Book of Experimental Psychology*, 2nd ed., 2 vols., 8vo, Cambridge 1911.

SANFORD, E. C., *A Course in Experimental Psychology*, Boston, 1898.

STERN, W., *Die differentielle Psychologie in ihren methodischen Grundlagen*, 3rd ed., 8vo, Leipzig, 1921.

TITCHENER, E. B., *Experimental Psychology. A Manual of Laboratory Practice*, 4 vols., 8vo, London and New York, 1901–5.

TOULOUSE, E. and PIÉRON, H., *Technique de Psychologie Expérimentale*, 2nd ed., 2 vols., 16mo, Paris, 1911.

WHIPPLE, G. M., *Manual of Mental and Physical Tests*, 3rd ed., 2 vols., 8vo, Baltimore, 1921.

4.—WORKS OF HISTORICAL AND DOCTRINAL INTEREST

BECHTEREW, W., *La Psychologie Objective*, trans. Kostyleff, 8vo, Paris, 1913.

BINET, A., *Introduction à la Psychologie Expérimentale*, 16mo, Paris, 1894.

FECHNER, G. T., *Elemente der Psychophysik* (1st ed. in 1859), 2nd ed., 2 vols., 8vo, Leipzig, 1889.

FOUCAULT, M., *La Psychophysique*, 8vo, Paris, 1901.

KANTOR, J. R., *Principles of Psychology*, 8vo, New York, 1924.

MCDOUGALL, W., *Psychology, the Study of Behaviour*, 16mo, London, 1912.

RIBOT, T., *English Psychology*, London, 1873, 2nd ed., 1892. *German Psychology of To-day*, New York, 1886, 2nd ed., London, 1892.

SCRIPTURE, E. W., *The New Psychology*, 8vo, London, 1897.

WARD, J., article " Psychology " in the *Encyclopædia Britannica*, 1886, republished as *Psychological Principles*, 8vo, Cambridge, 1918.

WATSON, J. B., *Psychology from the Standpoint of a Behaviorist*, 8vo, Philadelphia, 1919.

INDEX